Sodium Intake and Related Diseases

Sodium Intake and Related Diseases

Editors

Massimo Lucarini
Pasquale Strazzullo
Antonello Santini
Alessandra Durazzo
Ginevra Lombardi-Boccia
Stefania Sette

MDPI • Basel • Beijing • Wuhan • Barcelona • Belgrade • Manchester • Tokyo • Cluj • Tianjin

Editors

Massimo Lucarini
CREA-Research Centre for Food and Nutrition
Rome
Italy

Pasquale Strazzullo
Department of Internal Medicine
University of Naples Federico II
Naples
Italy

Antonello Santini
Department of Pharmacy
University of Napoli Federico II
Napoli
Italy

Alessandra Durazzo
CREA-Research Centre for Food and Nutrition
Rome
Italy

Ginevra Lombardi-Boccia
CREA-Research Centre for Food and Nutrition
Rome
Italy

Stefania Sette
CREA-Research Centre for Food and Nutrition
Rome
Italy

Editorial Office
MDPI
St. Alban-Anlage 66
4052 Basel, Switzerland

This is a reprint of articles from the Special Issue published online in the open access journal *International Journal of Molecular Sciences* (ISSN 1422-0067) (available at: www.mdpi.com/journal/ijms/special_issues/sodium_intake_diseases).

For citation purposes, cite each article independently as indicated on the article page online and as indicated below:

LastName, A.A.; LastName, B.B.; LastName, C.C. Article Title. *Journal Name* **Year**, *Volume Number*, Page Range.

ISBN 978-3-0365-1931-9 (Hbk)
ISBN 978-3-0365-1930-2 (PDF)

Contents

About the Editors

Massimo Lucarini

Massimo Lucarini holds a master's degree in Industrial Chemistry 'cum laude' at the University of Rome "La Sapienza", Italy (1992) and a Ph.D. in Chemistry (University of Rome "La Sapienza"). He works as researcher, at CREA, the Research Centre for Food and Nutrition (www.crea.gov.it). Here, research activity mainly aims to evaluate the nutrient contents of molecules with biological and anti-nutrient activity in foods and diets. An integral part of the research carried out is linked to institutional activity, including food composition tables, dietary guidelines for healthy eating, and evaluations of fraud risk in the agri-food system. The research activity also aims to exchange scientific information and acquire new skills both at national and international levels, through training courses and participation in congresses and seminars. The dissemination activity is carried out through the production of scientific articles and educational and informative activities.

Pasquale Strazzullo

Prof. Pasquale Strazzullo, MD, FAHA, is President of the Italian Society of Human Nutrition (SINU) and Associate Editor (past-Editor-in-chief) of *Nutrition, Metabolism and Cardiovascular Disease* (*NMCD*), the official journal of the Italian Societies of Human Nutrition, Diabetes and Atherosclerosis. He is the Italian Delegate in the WHO European Salt Action Network. Until last year, he was the Professor of Internal Medicine at Federico II University of Naples Medical School (Department of Clinical Medicine and Surgery), and has been Director of the Department of Clinica Medica as ESH Hypertension Specialist, responsible for the Excellence Centre of Hypertension. His broad areas of interest are the role of nutrition in cardiovascular prevention, the pathophysiology and clinical aspects of the disorders of mineral metabolism, and the metabolic and genetic bases of cardiovascular diseases. He has authored over 350 publications, most of which are in international, peer-reviewed journals.

Antonello Santini

Antonello Santini, Ph.D., is a Professor of Food Chemistry and Food Chemistry and Analysis of Food and Nutraceuticals at the Department of Pharmacy and at the Department of Agriculture of the University of Napoli Federico II, Napoli, Italy. He is also a visiting professor at the Albanian University of Tirana, Albania. He holds a Ph.D. in Chemical Sciences. His research areas of interest are substantiated by many international collaborations, mainly in the fields of food; food chemistry, nutraceuticals, and functional food; supplements; the recovery of natural compounds using eco-sustainable and environmentally friendly techniques from agro-food byproducts; nanocompounds; nanonutraceuticals; food risk assessments, safety and contaminants; mycotoxins and secondary metabolites; food analysis; and chemistry and food education. He is responsible for several funded research projects. His research activity is substantiated by more than 200 papers in internationally reputed, peer-reviewed journals.

Alessandra Durazzo

Alessandra Durazzo was awarded a master's degree in Chemistry and Pharmaceutical Technology cum laude in 2003, and a Ph.D. in Horticulture in 2010. She is a researcher at the CREA, Research Centre for Food and Nutrition. The core of her research is the study of chemical, nutritional and bioactive components of food, with particular regard to the wide spectrum of substance classes and their nutraceutical features. Her research activities also address the development, management and updating of bioactive compounds, nutraceuticals and dietary supplements databases; particular attention is given towards the harmonization of analytical procedures and the classification and codification of dietary supplements.

Ginevra Lombardi-Boccia

Ginevra Lombardi-Boccia graduated with a degree in Biological Science at the "La Sapienza" University of Rome. She is a senior Researcher at the Food Science Laboratories of CREA, Research Centre for Food and Nutrition. She is the co-author of more than 200 international peer-reviewed papers. She is also the Scientific Coordinator and co-leader of research projects aiming to assess the nutritional quality of food and diets and sustainability and innovation in food production. Her current research activities aim to identify and valorize new sustainable sources (e.g., food waste) of nutrients (e.g., proteins and omega3 fatty acids) and bioactive molecules (e.g., carotenoids and phenolics) and at recovering waste from food chains to develop products for the food, nutraceutical and cosmeceutical sectors.

Stefania Sette

Stefania Sette works at CREA, the Research Centre for Food and Nutrition. Her main scientific activities are: (i) food consumption studies and dietary assessments in Italy and developing countries; (ii) population and nationwide monitoring studies; (iii) nutritional research on food consumption pattern and factors affecting physical conditions; (iv) food preferences and school-meal surveys; (v) exposure assessments to chemicals, in particular, natural and artificial flavourings in foods; (vi) updates of food reference databases to be used in computer-based food systems to generate and process food consumption surveys; and (vii) research on aspects of food and nutrition policies.

International Journal of *Molecular Sciences*

MDPI

Editorial

Sodium Intake and Related Diseases

Massimo Lucarini [1,*], Alessandra Durazzo [1], Stefania Sette [1], Ginevra Lombardi-Boccia [1], Antonello Santini [2] and Pasquale Strazzullo [3,*]

1 CREA-Research Centre for Food and Nutrition, Via Ardeatina 546, 00178 Rome, Italy; alessandra.durazzo@crea.gov.it (A.D.); stefania.sette@crea.gov.it (S.S.); g.lombardiboccia@crea.gov.it (G.L.-B.)
2 Department of Pharmacy, University of Napoli Federico II, Via D. Montesano 49, 80131 Napoli, Italy; asantini@unina.it
3 Department of Clinical Medicine and Surgery, Federico II University of Naples, Via S. Pansini 5, 80131 Naples, Italy
* Correspondence: massimo.lucarini@crea.gov.it (M.L.); strazzul@unina.it (P.S.)

Citation: Lucarini, M.; Durazzo, A.; Sette, S.; Lombardi-Boccia, G.; Santini, A.; Strazzullo, P. Sodium Intake and Related Diseases. *Int. J. Mol. Sci.* **2021**, 22, 7608. https://doi.org/10.3390/ijms22147608

Received: 1 July 2021
Accepted: 12 July 2021
Published: 16 July 2021

Moderation in the use of salt (sodium chloride) in food and food preparations prevents the tendency of blood pressure to increase with age, and this is documented by many studies in current literature. In contrast, the abuse of salt frequently leads to increases in blood pressure and contributes to the development of hypertension, particularly in overweight or obese people, in diabetics, in the elderly and in genetically predisposed subjects.

Given the well-known relationship between high blood pressure and the risk of cardiovascular disease, high salt consumption is also associated with an increased risk of fatal or otherwise debilitating cardiovascular events, with a high impact on health expenditure.

The reduction of salt consumption leads to a decrease in blood pressure—more so in hypertensive, elderly and obese subjects—and consequently to a reduction in cardiovascular risk. The development of salt-reducing programs for individual, population, and country-level strategies to reduce salt intake is becoming a challenge, considering the general tendency not to change the use of salt. Improving knowledge is a key step for behavioral changes, suggesting the need for effective public health interventions throughout educational campaigns addressed at the implementation of good practices in nutrition [1,2].

The nutritional goal for the adult population has been set at no more than 2000 mg of sodium or 5 g of salt per day, in keeping with the WHO recommendation [3] that applies to all adult individuals, including the elderly, in the absence of different medical/nutritional indications.

At least half of the amount of salt taken individually comes from processed foods and food purchased and/or consumed outside of the home, and for these reasons an effective reduction in salt consumption requires the active participation of the food industry and the awareness of the consumer to the sodium content of the consumed products.

This Special Issue is focused on the role of sodium in the body's physiological processes. Generally, complex mechanisms regulate sodium concentrations in bodily fluids that involve the cardiovascular and endocrine systems, the central nervous system and the autonomic nervous system. The mechanisms involved in the regulation of sodium homeostasis will be the focus of this Special Issue. Some examples are the mechanisms which influence the action of the sodium–potassium pump, the renal tubular reabsorption mechanisms regulated by hormones, such as angiotensin II, and norepinephrine and those of sodium elimination, regulated by dopamine and cyclic AMP. The mechanisms involved at the molecular level of the relationship between sodium intake–blood pressure–cardiovascular disease and stomach cancer are among the focuses of this Special Issue.

The main topics of this Special Issue include: levels of intake and main sources of sodium from the diet: effect on the health status and description of the biochemical processes involved; salt intake and related risks; studies in the management and treatment of sodium intake-related diseases; epidemiological studies of the relationship between salt intake and related diseases: focus on the mechanism of action; delineation of mechanism of actions: *in vitro* and *in vivo* studies; salt and sapidity: mechanisms of taste perception. Chan et al. [4] investigated the MST3 involvement in Na^+ and K^+ homeostasis with increasing dietary potassium intake, in mice fed by diets containing various concentrations of Na^+ and K^+. The 2% KCl diets induced less MST3 expression in $MST3^{-/-}$ mice than that in wild-type (WT) mice. The $MST3^{-/-}$ mice had higher WNK4, NKCC2-S130 phosphorylation, and ENaC (epithelial Na channel) expression, resulting in lower urinary Na^+ and K^+ excretion than those of WT mice. Lower urinary Na^+ excretion was associated with elevated plasma $[Na^+]$ and hypertension. The authors marked how MST3 maintains Na^+/K^+ homeostasis in response to K^+ loading by regulation of WNK4 expression and NKCC2 and ENaC activity [4].

Hirohama et al. [5] showed, using animal models, how PGI2 analog attenuates salt-induced renal injury through the inhibition of inflammation and Rac1-MR activation; this study clearly demonstrated that Beraprost sodium (BPS), a pharmaceutical used in several Asian countries, including Japan and South Korea, as a vasodilator and antiplatelet agent, had renoprotective effects in salt-induced kidney injury, leading to the plausible hypothesis that BPS is therapeutically useful for the treatment of salt-induced renal damage.

Nakayama et al. [6] reported how Na^+ coupled nutrient cotransport-induced luminal negative potential and claudin-15 play an important role in paracellular Na^+ recycling in mouse small intestine; particularly, the authors concluded that Na^+, which is absorbed by Na^+-dependent glucose cotransport, is recycled back into the lumen via paracellular Na^+ conductance through claudin-15, which is driven by Na^+ cotransport induced luminal negativity [6].

It is worth mentioning the reviews by Patel and Joseph [7] on sodium intake and heart failure as well as that by Borrelli et al. [8] on sodium intake and chronic kidney disease.

This Special Issue contributes to the field of research on sodium, aiming to better understand its mechanism of action and reference and the relationship between sodium intake and related diseases.

Author Contributions: All the authors listed (M.L., A.D., S.S., G.L.-B., A.S. and P.S.) have made a substantial contribution to the work and approved it for publication. All authors have read and agreed to the published version of the manuscript.

Funding: This research received no external funding.

Acknowledgments: We would like to thank all the authors and the reviewers of the papers published in this Special Issue for their great contributions and efforts. We are also grateful to the editorial board members and to the staff of the journal for their kind support in all steps necessary for the realization of this Special Issue.

Conflicts of Interest: The authors declare no conflict of interest.

References

1. CREA–Research Centre for Food and Nutrition. Linee Guida per una Sana Alimentazione. Edizione. 2018. Available online: https://www.crea.gov.it/en/-/on-line-le-linee-guida-per-una-sana-alimentazione-2018 (accessed on 27 June 2021).
2. D'Elia, L.; La Fata, E.; Giaquinto, A.; Strazzullo, P.; Galletti, F. Effect of dietary salt restriction on central blood pressure: A systematic review and meta-analysis of the intervention studies. *J. Clin. Hypertens.* **2020**, *22*, 814–825. [CrossRef] [PubMed]
3. WHO Recommendation 2020. Available online: https://www.who.int/news-room/fact-sheets/detail/salt-reduction (accessed on 27 June 2021).
4. Chan, C.-H.; Wu, S.-N.; Bao, B.-Y.; Li, H.-W.; Lu, T.-L. MST3 Involvement in Na^+ and K^+ Homeostasis with Increasing Dietary Potassium Intake. *Int. J. Mol. Sci.* **2021**, *22*, 999. [CrossRef] [PubMed]
5. Hirohama, D.; Kawarazaki, W.; Nishimoto, M.; Ayuzawa, N.; Marumo, T.; Shibata, S.; Fujita, T. PGI_2 Analog Attenuates Salt-Induced Renal Injury through the Inhibition of Inflammation and Rac1-MR Activation. *Int. J. Mol. Sci.* **2020**, *21*, 4433. [CrossRef] [PubMed]
6. Nakayama, M.; Ishizuka, N.; Hempstock, W.; Ikari, A.; Hayashi, H. Na^+-Coupled Nutrient Cotransport Induced Luminal Negative Potential and Claudin-15 Play an Important Role in Paracellular Na^+ Recycling in Mouse Small Intestine. *Int. J. Mol. Sci.* **2020**, *21*, 376. [CrossRef] [PubMed]

7. Patel, Y.; Joseph, J. Sodium Intake and Heart Failure. *Int. J. Mol. Sci.* **2020**, *21*, 9474. [CrossRef] [PubMed]
8. Borrelli, S.; Provenzano, M.; Gagliardi, I.; Michael, A.; Liberti, M.E.; De Nicola, L.; Conte, G.; Garofalo, C.; Andreucci, M. Sodium Intake and Chronic Kidney Disease. *Int. J. Mol. Sci.* **2020**, *21*, 4744. [CrossRef] [PubMed]

International Journal of *Molecular Sciences*

MDPI

Article

MST3 Involvement in Na^+ and K^+ Homeostasis with Increasing Dietary Potassium Intake

Chee-Hong Chan [1], Sheng-Nan Wu [2], Bo-Ying Bao [3,4], Houng-Wei Li [5] and Te-Ling Lu [3,*]

1 Department of Nephrology, Chang Bing Show Chwan Memorial Hospital, Lukang, Changhua 505, Taiwan; cheehong.chan@gmail.com
2 Department of Physiology, National Cheng Kung University Medical College, Tainan 70101, Taiwan; snwu@mail.ncku.edu.tw
3 School of Pharmacy, China Medical University, Taichung 406040, Taiwan; bao@mail.cmu.edu.tw
4 Department of Nursing, Asia University, Taichung 41354, Taiwan
5 Department of Medical Laboratory Science and Biotechnology, China Medical University, Taichung 406040, Taiwan; albertli489@gmail.com
* Correspondence: lutl@mail.cmu.edu.tw

Abstract: K^+ loading inhibits NKCC2 (Na-K-Cl cotransporter) and NCC (Na-Cl cotransporter) in the early distal tubules, resulting in Na^+ delivery to the late distal convoluted tubules (DCTs). In the DCTs, Na^+ entry through ENaC (epithelial Na channel) drives K^+ secretion through ROMK (renal outer medullary potassium channel). WNK4 (with-no-lysine 4) regulates the NCC/NKCC2 through SAPK (Ste20-related proline-alanine-rich kinase)/OSR1 (oxidative stress responsive). K^+ loading increases intracellular Cl^-, which binds to the WNK4, thereby inhibiting autophosphorylation and downstream signals. Acute K^+ loading-deactivated NCC was not observed in Cl^--insensitive WNK4 mice, indicating that WNK4 was involved in K^+ loading-inhibited NCC activity. However, chronic K^+ loading deactivated NCC in Cl^--insensitive WNK4 mice, indicating that other mechanisms may be involved. We previously reported that mammalian Ste20-like protein kinase 3 (MST3/STK24) was expressed mainly in the medullary TAL (thick ascending tubule) and at lower levels in the DCTs. $MST3^{-/-}$ mice exhibited higher ENaC activity, causing hypernatremia and hypertension. To investigate MST3 function in maintaining Na^+/K^+ homeostasis in kidneys, mice were fed diets containing various concentrations of Na^+ and K^+. The 2% KCl diets induced less MST3 expression in $MST3^{-/-}$ mice than that in wild-type (WT) mice. The $MST3^{-/-}$ mice had higher WNK4, NKCC2-S130 phosphorylation, and ENaC expression, resulting in lower urinary Na^+ and K^+ excretion than those of WT mice. Lower urinary Na^+ excretion was associated with elevated plasma $[Na^+]$ and hypertension. These results suggest that MST3 maintains Na^+/K^+ homeostasis in response to K^+ loading by regulation of WNK4 expression and NKCC2 and ENaC activity.

Keywords: MST3; STK24; high potassium; ENaC; NKCC2; SPAK; OSR1; WNK4

Citation: Chan, C.-H.; Wu, S.-N.; Bao, B.-Y.; Li, H.-W.; Lu, T.-L. MST3 Involvement in Na^+ and K^+ Homeostasis with Increasing Dietary Potassium Intake. *Int. J. Mol. Sci.* **2021**, *22*, 999. https://doi.org/10.3390/ijms22030999

Academic Editor: Pasquale Strazzullo
Received: 15 December 2020
Accepted: 15 January 2021
Published: 20 January 2021

1. Introduction

An increase in dietary K^+ intake stimulates aldosterone release, which stimulates renal K^+ secretion, and does not influence Na^+ retention. Several Na^+ and K^+ channels coordinate to maintain K^+ secretion without Na^+ retention. The model of the process suggests that K^+ loading inhibits NKCC2 in the loop of Henle [1,2] and NCC activation [3,4], thus, the Na^+ is delivered to the distal nephron. The increased Na^+ in the distal nephron stimulates K^+ secretion through ROMK due to an electrochemical gradient generated by reabsorption of Na^+ through ENaC.

These channels are regulated by a group of serine/threonine kinases, WNKs. Mutations in WNK1 and WNK4 genes cause a hereditary disease known as pseudohypoaldosteronism type II (PHAII) characterized with hyperkalemic hypertension [5]. WNK4 is a physiological Cl^- sensor that manipulates dietary K^+ intake [6] and regulates NCC activation through downstream kinases SAPK and OSR1 [7]. Chloride efflux from the cells occurs in K^+ deficiency, resulting in low intracellular Cl^- ($[Cl^-]_i$) that stimulates WNK4 kinase, which phosphorylates SPAK and thus induces NCC phosphorylation [8,9]. The acute K^+ loading by oral gavage dephosphorylates NCC in wild-type (WT) mice after 30 min oral gavage of K^+. The decrease in phospho-NCC is not observed in the WNK4-Cl^- insensitive knock-in mice. These results indicated that high extracellular K^+ by increasing $[Cl^-]_i$ inhibits WNK4 and thus inactivates NCC [6]. Interestingly, long-term K^+ loading still dephosphorylates NCC in the WNK4-Cl^- insensitive knock-in mice, indicating that other molecules may be involved in HK-inhibited WNK4 and its downstream signaling [6].

WNK4 also modulates NKCC2 activity. NKCC2 abundance and NKCC2 activity are lower in WNK4$^{-/-}$ mice than that in controls [10]. Phosphorylation of NKCC2 is regulated by Ste-20 family kinases, including SPAK [11] and OSR1 [12]. SPAK mutant mice have a SPAK-activation deficiency, manifest reduced NKCC2 phosphorylation at T96, and are substantially hypotensive [13]. In addition to T96, NKCC2 overexpressed in the cells is phosphorylated at S91, T100, T105, and S130 by SPAK/OSR1 activation under hypotonic low-chloride conditions. Mutation of T105 or S130 reduces NKCC2 activity by 30–40% [14]. NKCC2 is known to account for approximately 20–25% of Na^+ reabsorption in the kidney [15], and phosphorylation of T105 and S130 plays the most important role in stimulation of NKCC2 activity. However, S130 phosphorylation has not been detected in the mouse kidney and the mechanism of regulation of phosphorylation of NKCC2 at S130 in vivo is unclear [14].

Na^+ delivered from K^+ loading-inhibited NCC and NKCC2 is reabsorbed through ENaC. Hence, K^+ loading induces ENaC expression and increases the channel activity to prevent Na^+ loss. ENaC is composed of the α, β, and γ subunits, which are delivered to the apical surface after the synthesis. The activity of ENaC at the apical surface is regulated by proteases, which cleave the α- and γ-ENaC subunits to increase open probability of the channel [16]. An increase in dietary K^+ intake significantly increased both ENaC and ROMK currents; however, K^+ loading-induced stimulation of Na^+ and K^+ currents was smaller in mice carrying PHAII-mimicking mutations [17]. These results indicate that molecules downstream of WNK4 may be involved in K^+ loading-regulated ENaC and ROMK activity.

We found that MST3 expression is higher in the medullary thick ascending limb (TAL) than that in the distal convoluted tubules (DCTs) in mice [18], and MST3 protects MDCK cells from physiological hypertonic stress in vitro [19]. To investigate whether MST3 was involved in ion homeostasis, we generated MST3-targeted mutant mice. Since complete knockout of MST3 was not achievable, we reported the phenotype of MST3 hypomorphic mice (referred to as MST3$^{-/-}$ mice) that manifested enhanced ENaC activity and hypertension [18]. These results indicated that MST3, similar to other Ste20 family members, played an important role in the maintenance of Na^+ homeostasis. In the present study, we investigated whether MST3 was involved in the regulation of Na^+ and K^+ homeostasis in response to K^+ loading. The expression levels of WNK4, ROMK, BK, ENaC, NCC, and NKCC2 were determined in mice fed the control and HK diets. Plasma Na^+ and urinary Na^+/K^+ excretion were also assayed.

2. Results

2.1. An Increase in MST3 Levels in Mouse Kidneys with Increasing K^+ Intake

Since we previously reported that MST3$^{-/-}$ mice have higher ENaC activity [18], we hypothesized that MST3$^{-/-}$ mice have higher ability to reabsorb Na^+ with a low-Na (LNa, 0.04% Na) diet challenge. To preserve Na^+ in Na^+ deficiency, WT (MST3$^{+/+}$) mice reduced urinary Na^+ excretion from 782.62 ± 152.57 to 90.89 ± 61.78 µmol/day (Figure 1A,B) and reduced urine volume from 5345.00 ± 861.55 to 3748.67 ± 789.03 µL/day (Figure 1C,D). MST3$^{-/-}$ mice also preserved Na^+ through a reduction in urinary Na^+ excretion from 589.13 ± 90.61 to 61.78 ± 22.26 µmol/day (Figure 1A,B) and urine volume from 3958.00 ± 1047.19 to 2729.31 ± 861.14 µL/day (Figure 1C,D). The urinary Na^+ excretion ratio of low Na (LNa) to control diets was 12.11 ± 3.8% in WT mice and

10.42 ± 2.7% in MST3$^{-/-}$ mice. The urine volume ratio of LNa to control diets was 70.58 ± 13.19% in WT mice and 67.55 ± 12.91% in MST3$^{-/-}$ mice. There were no differences between WT and MST3$^{-/-}$ mice in Na^+ reabsorption in Na^+ deficiency. However, we previously reported that MST3 protein level is upregulated in WT mice after high-salt (HS) intake (8% Na, 1.1% K) [19]. The HS diet-fed mice intake two-fold higher levels of water and chow than those animals fed the control diets (Table 1), indicating that the animals intake higher levels of both Na^+ and K^+. To investigate the effects of Na^+ or K^+ separately, we fed mice with increasing Na^+ and increasing K^+ by adding 1% NaCl and 1% KCl in drinking water to determine the effects of Na^+ and K^+ on MST3. The MST3 expression was similar in kidney to that of control, LNa or 1.43% Na diet (0.43% Na in chow with additional 1% NaCl in drinking water) (Figure 2A). Interestingly, 2% KCl (1% K in chow with additional 1% KCl in drinking water) stimulated MST3 expression (Figure 2B). To determine the effect of K^+-loading on MST3 function in the kidney, we fed WT and MST3$^{-/-}$ mice 2% KCl diets. The 2% KCl diets stimulated an approximately 1.6-fold increase in MST3 expression in WT mice (Figure 2C, lanes 4–6). MST3$^{-/-}$ mice consistently expressed a lower level of MST3 than that in WT mice (Figure 2C, lanes 7–9); however, we observed only a 1.1-fold increase in MST3 expression in 2% KCl diet-fed MST3$^{-/-}$ mice (Figure 2C, lanes 10–12).

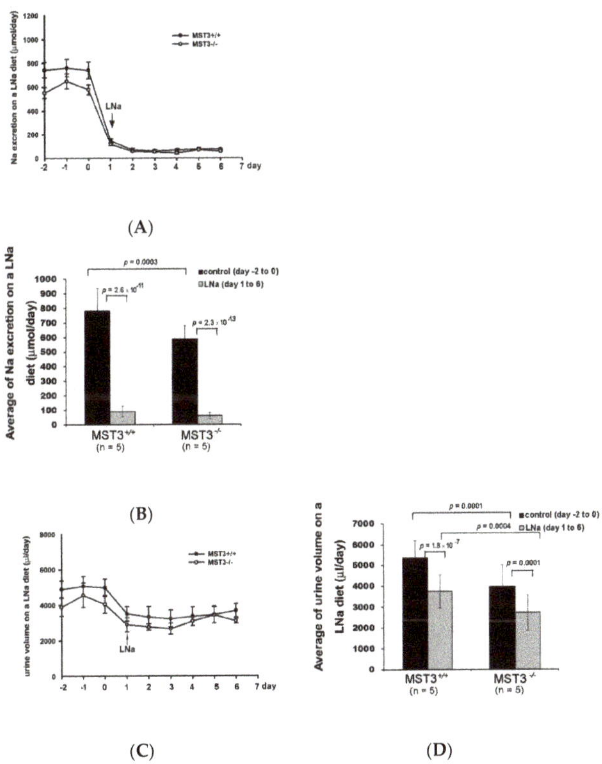

Figure 1. Urinary Na^+ excretion and urine volume on a low Na (LNa) diet. Wild-type (WT) (MST$^{+/+}$) (•) and MST3$^{-/-}$ (○) mice were fed the control diet for 3 days; then, the diet was changed to the LNa diet for an additional 16 days. The average group values were used to generate the graphs, and the error bars correspond to SE. Urinary Na^+ excretion (**A**) and urine volume (**C**) were recorded over 9 days. The bar graphs (**B**,**D**) show the average of the data in (**A**,**C**), respectively.

Table 1. The values of weight, water intake, and food intake in 8-week-old C57Bl/6 male mice fed control or high salt diets.

Diet	Control Diet (0.43% Na, 1.1% K) (n = 5)	High Salt (8% Na, 1.1% K) (n = 5)
Weight, g	19.55 ± 2.12	21.94 ± 1.52
Water intake, mL	4.96 ± 0.52	8.62 ± 1.01
Food intake, g	3.17 ± 0.43	8.82 ± 1.89

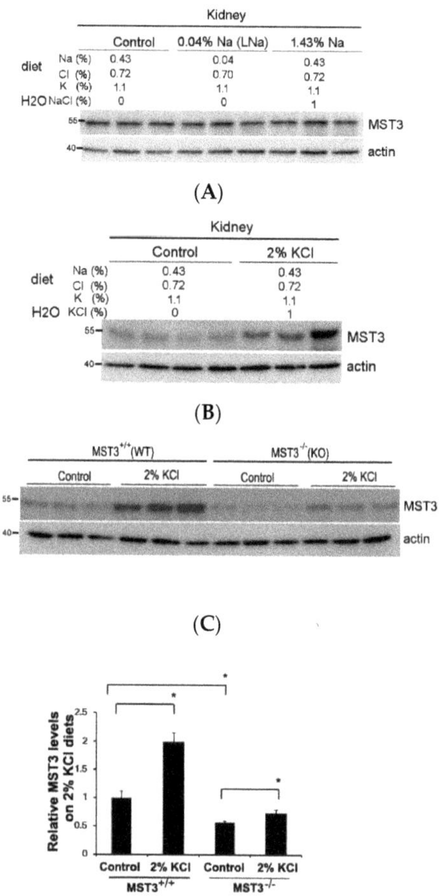

Figure 2. A 2% KCl diet stimulates MST3 expression. MST3 protein expression was detected in WT mice fed the (**A**) control (n = 3 or 4 animals), low Na (LNa), 1.43% Na or (**B**) 2% KCl diets for 16 days (n = 3 animals/group). The sodium, potassium, chloride and water contents in the diet are indicated. (**C**) MST3 protein expression was detected in WT and MST3$^{-/-}$ mice fed the control and 2% KCl diets (n = 3 animals/group). (**D**) The bar graph shows quantification of MST3 expression in (**C**). * $p < 0.05$ vs. the control group.

2.2. Reduction of Diuresis, Kaliuresis, and Natriuresis in MST3$^{-/-}$ Mice Fed 2% KCl Diets

Consistent with the notion that K^+ loading causes diuresis and kaliuresis [20], K^+ loading induced a rapid diuresis in WT mice (urine volume from 4812.22 ± 695.51 to 5700.80 ± 792.40 μL) on day 1 of K^+ loading and remained at 6813.83 ± 2229.64 μL during days 2–6 of K^+ loading. However, the urine volume of MST3$^{-/-}$ mice was increased only from 3884.58 ± 695.51 to 5875.00 ± 993.79 μL on day 1 of K^+ loading and was reduced to 3652.50 ± 893.94 μL on subsequent days of K^+ loading (Figure 3A,B). A kaliuresis was also observed from 1082.92 ± 136.58 to 1692.90 ± 136.58 μmol on day 1 of K^+ loading and remained at 1903.83 ± 435.69 μmol/d in WT mice (Figure 3C,D). These results indicated that in response to increasing K^+ intake, the kidneys normally excreted approximately 1.75-fold of K^+, which was between 90 to 95% of the daily 2-fold increase of K^+ intake (Figure 3D); however, urinary K^+ excretion in MST3$^{-/-}$ mice was substantially increased from 948.49 ± 105.69 to 1873.12 ± 370.63 μL on day 1 of K^+ loading and was then slightly increased to 1230.35 ± 205.69 μL (Figure 3C,D). Comparison of the fold change of the urine volume on K^+ loading to the control diets indicated an approximately 1.4-fold increase after K^+ loading in WT mice. The urine volume in K^+ loading-treated MST3$^{-/-}$ mice was only 0.8-fold of that in control diet-fed mice, significantly less than the 1.4-fold increase in WT mice ($p = 1.8 \times 10^{-5}$) (Figure 3). When comparing the fold change of K^+ secretion on K^+ loading, only a 1.29-fold increase was detected in MST3$^{-/-}$ mice, which was significantly less than a 1.75-fold increase in WT mice ($p = 4.0 \times 10^{-6}$) (Figure 3D), indicating that MST3$^{-/-}$ mice exhibited reduced diuresis and kaliuresis than that in WT mice on K^+ loading.

The urinary Na^+ excretion in WT mice was slightly reduced from 763.10 ± 87.68 to 680.59 ± 44.45 μmol on day 1 of K^+ loading and returned back to 712.87 ± 102.34 μmol/d on subsequent days of K^+ loading, indicating that Na^+ was maintained at homeostasis. In contrast, urinary Na^+ excretion was significantly decreased in MST3$^{-/-}$ mice from 663.74 ± 79.60 to 532.68 ± 71.95 μmol after K^+ loading (Figure 3E,F) and reduced to approximately 0.8-fold of that in mice fed control diet; these levels were significantly less than those in WT mice (0.93-fold change, $p = 0.0006$) (Figure 3F). These results indicated that MST3$^{-/-}$ mice reabsorbed higher amounts of Na^+ and water than those in WT mice on 2% KCl diets. This increase in Na^+ reabsorption was associated with an increase in the plasma [Na^+] (in mM, 154.67 in MST3$^{-/-}$ mice vs. 152.5 in MST3$^{+/+}$ mice) (Table 2). Overall, the Na^+- and flow-dependent K^+ secretion was inhibited in MST3$^{-/-}$ mice. After K^+ loading, systolic blood pressure (SBP) of WT mice was 119 ± 10 mm Hg, which was similar to the SBP in mice fed the control diet; however, SBP of MST3$^{-/-}$ mice was 131 ± 9 mm Hg (Table 2). These results suggested that only a 1.1-fold increase in MST3 in MST3$^{-/-}$ mice fed the 2% KCl diets was insufficient to excrete Na^+ and K^+, causing elevated SBP in MST3$^{-/-}$ mice.

Table 2. Blood pressure (BP) in WT and MST3$^{-/-}$ mice on control diets for 3 days and challenged with 2% KCl diets. * $p < 0.05$ vs. the WT group.

		Value	
	16 Days	**MST3$^{+/+}$ (WT)**	**MST3$^{-/-}$**
Plasma [Na^+] (mmol/L)	control diet	152.33 ± 0.52	153.4 ± 0.89 *
	2% KCl diets	152.5 ± 0.84	154.67 ± 1.53 *
Blood pressure (mmHg)	control diet	117 ± 9	130 ± 13 *
	2% KCl diets	118 ± 10	131 ± 9 *

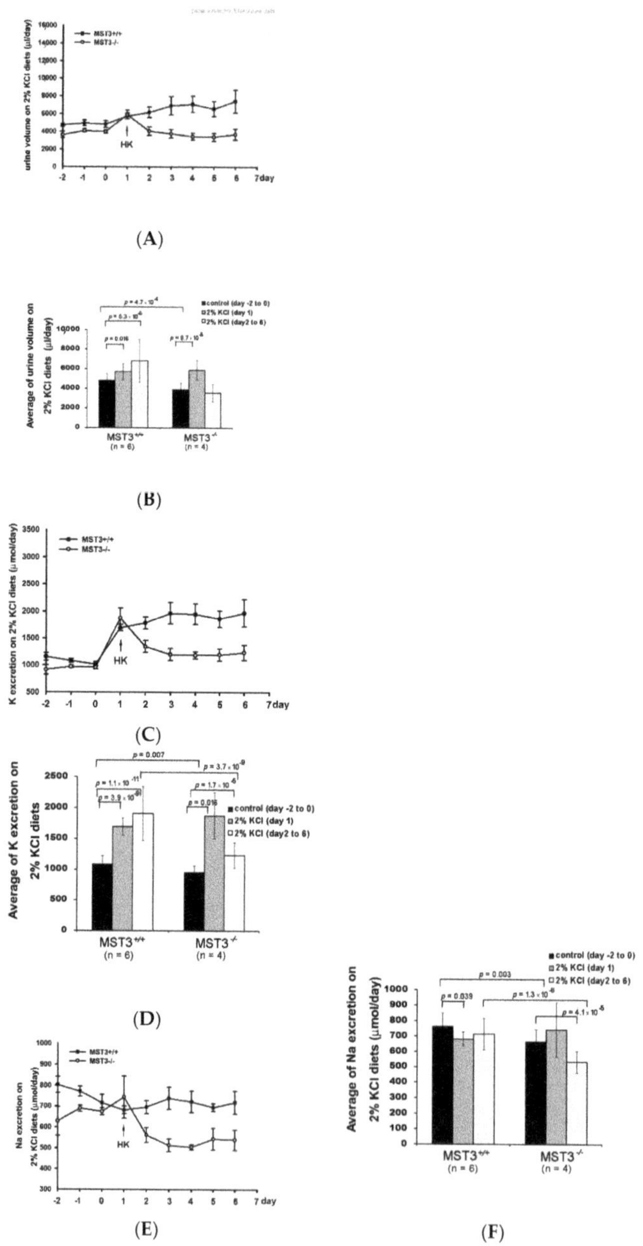

Figure 3. Reduction of diuresis, kaliuresis, and natriuresis in $MST3^{-/-}$ mice fed 2% KCl diets. $MST^{+/+}$ (●) and $MST3^{-/-}$ (○) mice were fed a control diet for 3 days; then, the diet was changed to the 2% KCl diet for an additional 16 days. The urine volume (**A**), urinary K^+ (**C**), and urinary Na^+ (**E**) excretion were recorded over 9 days. The average group values were used to generate the graphs, and the error bars correspond to SE. The bar graphs (**B**,**D**,**F**) show the average of the data in (**A**,**C**,**E**) respectively.

2.3. WNK4 and WNK4-Regulated Channels in 2% KCl Diet-Fed Mice

WNK4 plays an important role in modulating renal K^+ secretion and Na^+ absorption. We found that 2% KCl diets induced increased WNK4 expression in $MST3^{-/-}$ mice (Figure 4A), indicating that MST3 might be involved in WNK4 regulation. WNK4 have been shown to inhibit ROMK activity by stimulating clathrin-mediated endocytosis [21] and inhibiting maxi-K by a kinase-dependent mechanism [22]. Figure 4B showed that BK and ROMK were increased after K^+ loading in WT mice. In $MST3^{-/-}$ mice, there was no obvious difference in BK expression; however, ROMK was not induced after K^+ loading, which may cause reduced kaliuresis.

Consistent with the notion that K^+ loading induced ENaC γ-cleavage [6], 2% KCl diets induced increased cleaved γ-ENaC expression in WT mice, indicating that 2% KCl diets increased ENaC activity. Compared with WT mice, $MST3^{-/-}$ mice had a higher cleaved γ-ENaC on control diets and higher full-length ENaC on 2% KCl diets (Figure 4C). IHC results showed that feeding the 2% KCl diets slightly increased γ-ENaC expression at the apical plasma membrane of the DCT2/CNT in WT mice compared with that in mice fed the control diets (Figure 4D, c vs. a). Consistent with our previous report, $MST3^{-/-}$ mice exhibited higher ENaC expression at the apical plasma membrane of the DCT2/CNT. A higher intensity of ENaC staining was observed on 2% KCl diets (Figure 4D, g vs. e). The MST3 expression showed that higher levels of MST3 protein were present in the cytosol of the DCT2/CNT in WT mice on 2% KCl diets compared to that in WT mice on control diets (Figure 4D, d vs. b). Lower levels of MST3 were observed in $MST3^{-/-}$ mice on 2% KCl diets (Figure 4D, h).

Isoforms A, B, and F of NKCC2 are estimated to account for 20–25% of all renal Na^+ reabsorption. The NKCC2-F isoform mainly located in the inner medullary TAL accounts for 70% of NKCC2 expression [23]. Since MST3 is primarily localized in the inner medullary TAL, we determined whether MST3 is involved in K^+ loading-mediated NKCC2 phosphorylation. K^+ loading inhibited nonglycosylated NKCC2 phosphorylation at S130 in WT mice; however, the level of nonglycosylated and glycosylated phospho-S130-NKCC2 was increased in $MST3^{-/-}$ mice on 2% KCl diets (Figure 4E). These results indicated that MST3 inhibited NKCC2F phosphorylation at S130. IHC results showed that both MST3 (Figure 4F, G, b) and NKCC2 (Figure 4F, G, a) are mainly expressed at the apical membrane of the inner medullary TAL in control diet-fed WT mice. A 2% KCl diet induced MST3 expression ((Figure 4F, G, d) in the cytosol of the inner medullary TAL. NKCC2 was present at the subapical membrane of the inner medullary TAL (Figure 4F, G, c vs. a). This pattern is more clearly observed in an enlarged image (Figure 4G). However, in 2% KCl diet-fed $MST3^{-/-}$ mice, low levels of MST3 and higher levels of NKCC2 were still present at the apical membrane of the inner medullary TAL ((Figure 4F, 4G, g and h). These results indicated that MST3 inhibited medullary NKCC2 expression at the apical membrane of the medullary TAL in mice fed the 2% KCl diets.

The 2% KCl diets reduced the level of NCC in $MST3^{+/+}$ and $MST3^{-/-}$ mice (Figure 4H, lower panel), indicating that K^+ loading-inhibited NCC expression promoted K^+ secretion. However, there were no differences in phospho-NCC levels in $MST3^{+/+}$ and $MST3^{-/-}$ mice fed the 2% KCl diets (Figure 4H, upper panel). Additionally, there were no differences in the NCC distribution in the DCT1 in mice fed the control and 2% KCl diets (Figure 4I). These results indicated that MST3 may have a small or no effect on K^+ loading-mediated inhibition of NCC activity.

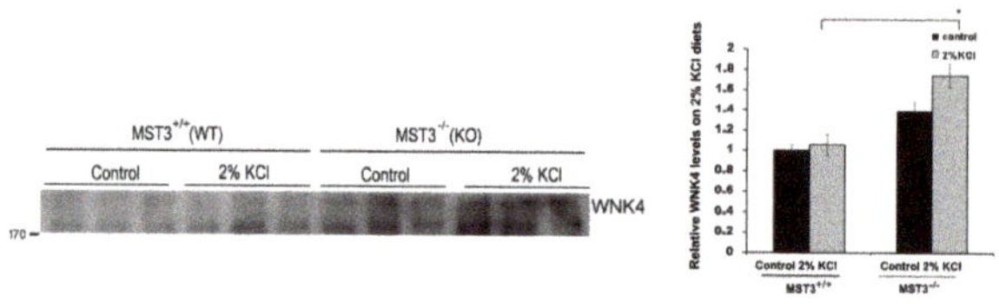

(**A**)

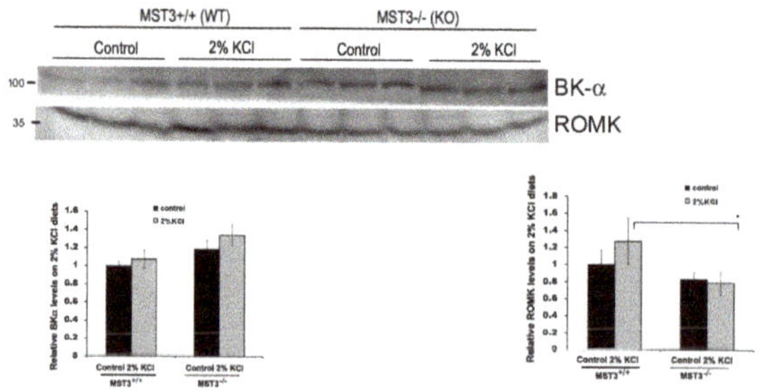

(**B**)

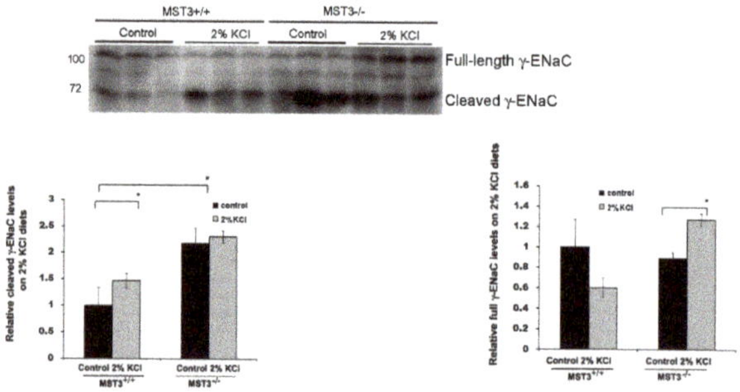

(**C**)

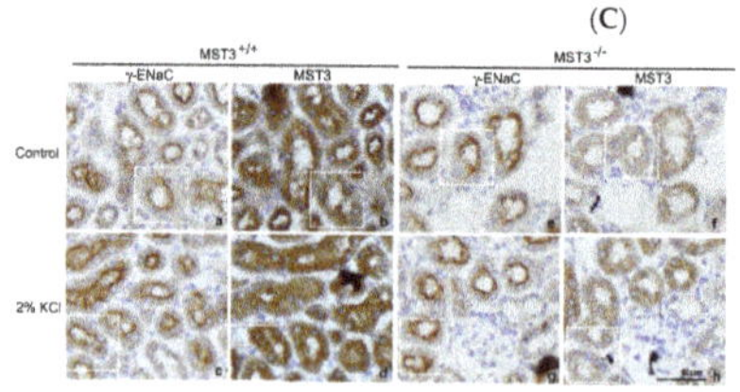

(**D**)

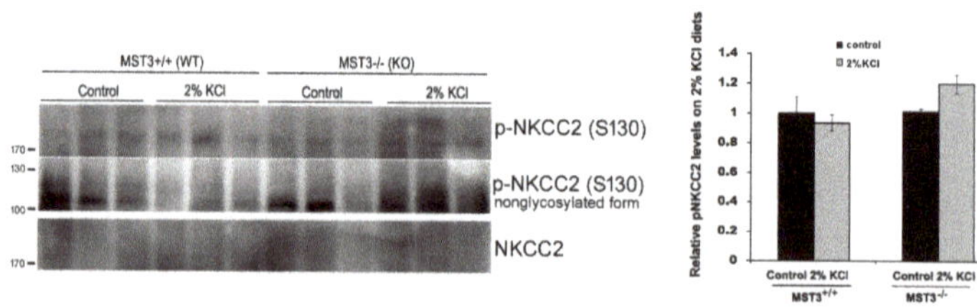

(**E**)

Figure 4. *Cont.*

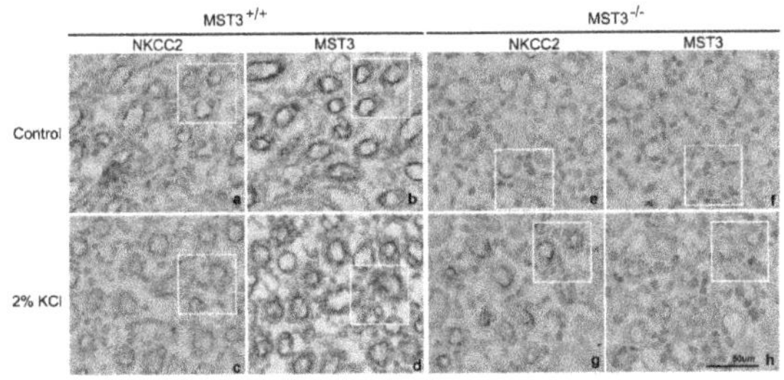

(F)

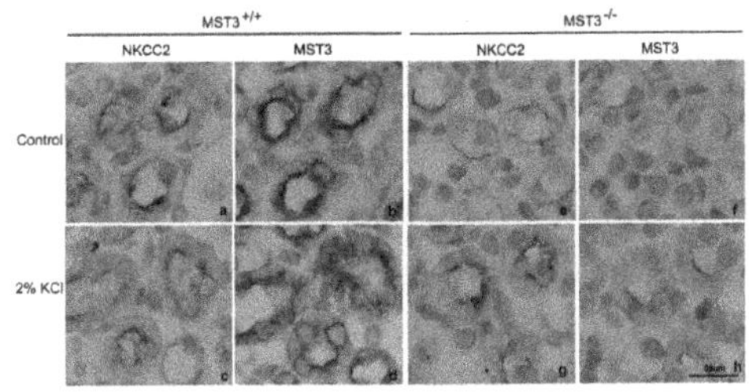

(G)

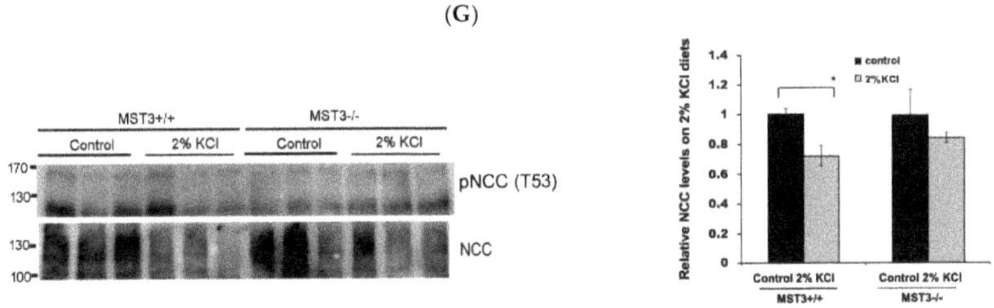

(H)

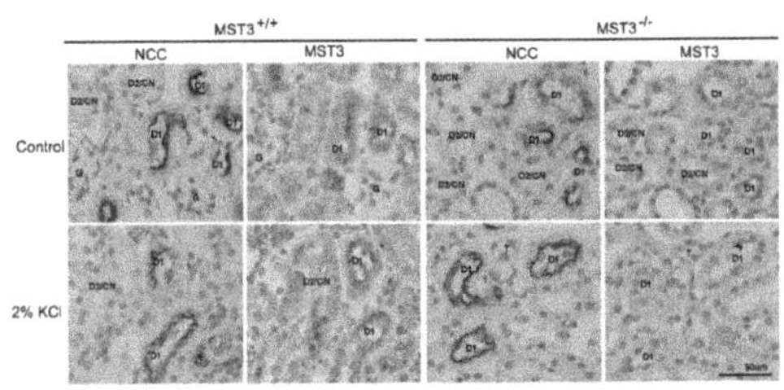

(I)

Figure 4. WNK4 and WNK4-regulated channels in mice fed 2% KCl diets. Western blot analysis of (**A**) WNK4, (**B**) BK, and ROMK, (**C**) γ-ENaC, (**E**) NKCC2, and p-NKCC2, and (**H**) NCC and p-NCC in the kidney of MST$^{+/+}$ and MST3$^{-/-}$ mice 8 weeks after the treatment with the control and 2% KCl diets for 16 days (n = 3 animals/group). The bar graph shows quantification of Western blot relative to the levels in the control group of WT mice. * $p < 0.05$ vs. the control group. Serial sections of the kidney of WT and MST3$^{-/-}$ mice fed the control and 2% KCl diets were stained for γ-ENaC (**D**), NKCC2 (**F**,**G**, outlined images of **F** were enlarged using a 100× objective.), NCC (**I**), and MST3. G, glomerular; D1, early distal convoluted tubule; D2, late distal convoluted tubule; CN, connecting tubule.

3. Discussion

K^+ preferentially leaves the cells through K^+ channels, such as ROMK and BK, at the apical membrane of the DCT2/CNT. This process is driven by an electrochemical gradient generated by reabsorption of Na^+ through ENaC to induce a K^+-secreting state. Na^+ delivered to DCT2/CNT is due to K^+ loading-induced NCC and NKCC2 inhibition; thus, K^+ loading-inhibited NCC and NKCC2 and K^+ loading-induced ENaC activation needs to be strictly regulated to maintain Na^+ homeostasis (Figure 5). We found that the 2% KCl diets induced higher MST3 expression in WT mice than that in MST3$^{-/-}$ mice. MST3$^{-/-}$ mice with reduced MST3 expression had higher WNK4 expression, which might be involved in ENaC activity and NKCC2 phosphorylation at S130. These results indicated that MST3$^{-/-}$ mice reabsorbed more Na^+ at TAL, thus reducing K^+ secretion. In DCT2/CNT, MST3$^{-/-}$ mice had higher ENaC activity than that in WT mice, indicating that MST3$^{-/-}$ mice could not inhibit ENaC activation to prevent ENaC overactivation. Overall, MST3$^{-/-}$ mice reabsorbed more Na^+ and K^+ than did WT mice on HK diets. Our results indicate that MST3 functions to maintain Na^+ and K^+ homeostasis in mice on 2% KCl diets in vivo.

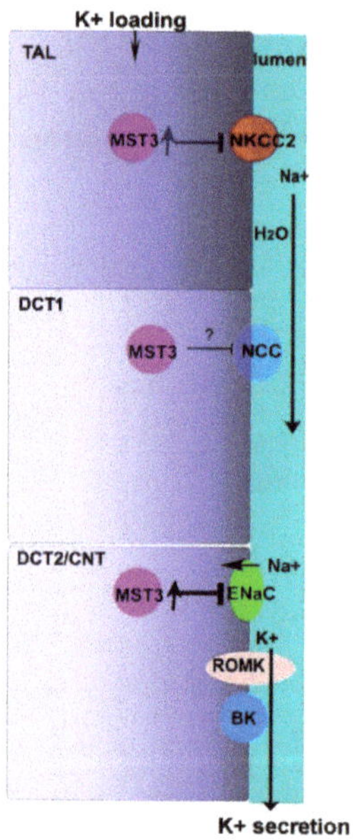

Figure 5. Hypothetical model of MST3 function on 2% KCl diets. NKCC2 and NCC in TAL and DCT1, respectively, are inhibited upon an increase in K^+ intake, thus, delivering Na^+ and water to the DCT2/CNT. Na^+ in the DCT2/CNT is reabsorbed through ENaC, resulting in K^+ secretion due to an electrochemical gradient. Reabsorption of Na^+ through ENaC at the DCT2/CNT prevents Na^+ loss. An increase in K^+ intake stimulates MST3 expression, which inhibits NKCC2 and ENaC expression at the apical membrane of the nephron, thus preventing excessive absorption of Na^+ and maintaining Na^+ homeostasis.

K^+ loading induces an increase in the circulating plasma levels of aldosterone to stimulate K^+ secretion, and then aldosterone has a smaller increase for longer periods [24]. In addition, HK-induced K^+ secretion is dependent on Na^+ delivery and flow, resulting from inhibition of Na^+ reabsorption in the TAL and DCT1. The resultant Na^+ delivery and flow along with increased aldosterone facilitate renal K^+ excretion through ROMK and BK channels [25–27]. Our results indicated that both WT and MST3$^{-/-}$ mice exhibited apid diuresis and kaliuresis on the 1st day K^+ loading; however, MST3$^{-/-}$ mice could not continually increase K^+ secretion on the subsequent days of HK challenge (Figure 3). We suggested that aldosterone might be involved in K^+ secretion at the beginning of the K^+ challenge, and then MST3 plays a role in Na^+-dependent and flow-dependent K^+ secretion.

Most studies used 5% K^+ in an HK diet; feeding this diet decreased the abundance of both NCC and phospho-NCC [6,8]. However, 5% K^+ is unphysiological. Modest changes in dietary K^+ affect plasma [K^+] and NCC in a graded manner [8]. We fed mice with modest changes of K^+ by increasing K^+ from 1% (1% in chow) to 2% K^+ (1% in chow and 1% in drinking water). An approximately 2-fold increase of urinary K^+ was excreted in response to increased K^+ intake (from 1% to 2%). The abundance of NCC was reduced in both MST3$^{+/+}$ and MST3$^{-/-}$ mice, indicating that NCC was inhibited, thus promoting K^+ secretion (Figure 4H, lower panel); however, phospho-NCC was not obviously inhibited (Figure 4H, upper panel), which may be due to the modest K^+ challenge in mice in the present study. The results of IHC analysis showed a lack of differences in NCC distribution in MST3$^{+/+}$ and MST3$^{-/-}$ mice (Figure 4I). These results suggested that the lowest MST3 expression in the DCT1 was not involved in 2% KCl loading-inhibited NCC activation in vivo.

WNK4 kinase activity is regulated by different mechanisms to transduce signals to downstream molecules. The KLHL3/CUL3 ubiquitin ligase complex degrades WNK4. In PHAII, the loss of interaction between KLHL3 and WNK4 increases levels of WNK4 [28]. Phosphorylation of WNK4 by PKC and PKA regulate the WNK4's activity and downstream signaling [29]. Protein phosphatase 1 binds to WNK4 and modulates the inhibitory effect of WNK4 on ROMK [30], and activation of protein phosphatases (PPs) may mediate NCC dephosphorylation in response to high extracellular K^+ [31]. In addition, WNK4 is a Cl^- sensor. WNK4 regulates WNK4 activity by binding to Cl^-. A WNK Cl^--sensing mechanism explains WNK-mediated regulation of NCC/NKCC2 by diets with various levels of K^+. At high intracellular chloride concentrations ($[Cl^-]_i$), chloride ions binds to WNK4, thus inhibiting WNK4 activity. The acute K^+ loading-dephosphorylated NCC was not observed in the WNK4-Cl^- insensitive knock-in mice, indicating that high extracellular K^+ by increasing $[Cl^-]_i$ inhibits WNK4 and thus inactivates NCC [6]. However, the long-term K^+ loading still dephosphorylates NCC in the WNK4-Cl^- insensitive knock-in mice, indicating that another mechanism was involved in HK-inhibited WNK4 and its downstream signaling. MST3$^{-/-}$ mice exhibited higher WNK4 expression (Figure 4A), higher ENaC activity (Figure 4C,D), and higher p-NKCC2 (Figure 4E,G) on 2% KCl diets for 16 days, indicating that MST3 was involved in WNK4 and its downstream signals. We have previously reported that MST3 was phosphorylated at the tyrosine residues. Tyrosine phosphorylation of MST3 may create a docking site for molecules involved in diverse signaling pathways [32]. We demonstrated that MST3 inhibited protein tyrosine phosphatase activity to inhibit cell migration through paxillin regulation [33]. Involvement of MST3 in phosphatase activity, ubiquitination, or WNK4 phosphorylation, which regulates ENaC activity and NKCC2 phosphorylation in the case of long-term K^+ loading, requires additional investigation.

Dietary potassium inhibits NCC- and NKCC2-mediated Na^+ reabsorption and shifts Na^+ downstream for reabsorption by ENaC, which can drive K^+ secretion and prevent Na^+ loss. This study reports that increased K^+ intake stimulates MST3 expression to inhibit Na^+ reabsorption. This effect is mediated by inhibition of NKCC2 and ENaC; inhibition of NKCC2 inhibits Na^+ reabsorption and promotes K^+ secretion; inhibition of ENaC does not increase Na^+ reabsorption, thus maintaining Na^+ homeostasis (Figure 5).

4. Methods

4.1. Animals

This study was approved by the Committee on the Ethics of Animal Experiments and was performed according to the Guidelines for Animal Experiments of the China Medical University (#CMUIACUC-2019-284-1; approved July 2019). C57BL/6 male mice in Table 1 were 12-weeks-old and housed in metabolic cages and allowed ad libitum access to food and water for 4 weeks [19]; the animals were divided into two groups: the control diet group (diets: 0.43% Na and 1.1% K (*w/w*)) and high-salt (HS) diet group (diets: 8% Na and 1.1% K (*w/w*); TestDiet, St. Louis, MO, USA). MST3$^{+/+}$ (WT) and MST3 hypomorphic mutant (designated MST3$^{-/-}$) mice were obtained as reported previously [18]. To investigate the effect of an increase in Na^+ or K^+ separately, we added additional 1% NaCl and 1% KCl into drinking water to make sure that the mice took in additional Na^+ and K^+. The mice were fed control, low Na (LNa), 1.43% Na (0.43% Na in chow with additional 1% NaCl in drinking water), and 2% KCl (1% K in chow with additional 1% KCl in drinking water) diet. Male WT and MST3$^{-/-}$ mice (8–12-weeks-old) were allowed ad libitum access to food and water. The mice were kept in metabolic cages, fed the control diet for the first 3 days and then challenged with LNa and HK diets for the following 6 days. Urine was collected during this period. Then, the animals were moved to the mouse cages and exposed to the corresponding challenge diet for the next 10 days.

4.2. Immunohistochemistry

The procedures have been described previously in detail. Briefly, serial sections of mouse kidneys were deparaffinized in xylene before rehydration in a graded series of ethanol and then the sample was incubated in a buffer (1 mM Tris in PBS, pH 8.2) at 100 °C for 20 min for antigens retrieval. Serial sections were incubated with antibodies against MST3 (1:500, a gift from Dr. Ming-Derg Lai, Taiwan), γ-ENaC (1:200, cat. no. 13943-1-AP; Proteintech, IL, USA), NCC (1:8000, cat. no. ab3553; Millipore, MA, USA), and NKCC2 (1:200, cat. no. AF2850; R&D Systems, MN, USA). Specificity of the anti-MST3 antibody was confirmed as previously report [18,33,34]. The secondary antibodies (1:1000, cat. no. 111-035-144; Jackson ImmunoResearch, PA, USA) were incubated at room temperature for 1 h with subsequent 3,3′-diaminobenzidine (DAB) (DAKO, Denmark, Hilden, Germany) staining.

4.3. Immunoblotting

Kidneys harvested from mice were homogenized using a PT 2100 Polytron homogenizer in ice-cold lysis solution containing 50 mM HEPES, pH 7.2, 150 mM NaCl, 1% Triton X-100, and protease inhibitors. The lysate from the kidney was first centrifuged at 100,000× *g* for 30 min at 4 °C. Samples from the supernatant were resolved by SDS-PAGE and transferred to NC paper. Western blot analysis was performed as reported previously [18] using primary antibodies against MST3 (1:1000), WNK4 (1:1000, cat. no. 22326-1-AP; Proteintech,, IL, USA), BKα (1:500, cat. no. APC-151; Alomone labs, Jerusalem, IL), ROMK (1:500, cat. no. APC-001; Alomone labs, Jerusalem, IL), γ-ENaC (1:1000), NCC (1:500), NKCC2 (1:1000), phospho-T53-NCC (1:500, cat. no. ab254039; Abcam, Cambridge, UK), and phospho-S130-NKCC2 (1:500, a gift from Dr. Dario Alessi, UK).

4.4. Measurement of Blood Pressure, Serum Na^+, and Urinary Concentrations of Na^+ and K^+ and Statistical Analysis

The steady-state SBP (systolic blood pressure) of restrained conscious mice was measured by a programmable tail-cuff sphygmomanometer (MK-2000ST, Muromachi, Tokyo, JP). SBP was initially estimated by inflating the cuff at approximately 25 mm Hg/sec. SBP was accurately determined during cuff deflation at approximately 4–5 mm Hg/sec. SBP was defined as blood pressure (BP) corresponding to the reappearance of the pulse. Blood samples were obtained via cheek pouch bleeding. Urine was collected from the urine collection tubes of the metabolic cages every 24 h for 9 days. The concentrations of Na^+ and K^+ were measured using an Advia 1800 chemistry system (Siemens). The levels of Na^+ and K^+ in urine and urine volume are shown as the mean ± SD. The statistical analysis was performed using Microsoft Excel 2013 by one-way analysis of variance (ANOVA) followed by Bonferroni post hoc tests. *p*-values *<0.05, **<0.005, and ***<0.0005 were considered significant. The mean values of the animals fed the control diet were averaged for the first 3 days of the treatment.

Author Contributions: C.-H.C. was responsible for experiment design, data collection and discussion. S.-N.W. contributed to experiments and discussion. B.-Y.B. was responsible for data collection and statistical analysis. H.-W.L. contributed to experiments and material preparation. T.-L.L. was responsible for writing, experimental design and materials. All authors have read and agreed to the published version of the manuscript.

Funding: This study was supported by the research grant MOST 108-2635-B-039-001 from the National Science Council of Taiwan, in part by grant CMU109-MF-89 from the China Medical University, Taiwan, and grant RD108006 from Chang Bing Show-Chwan Memorial Hospital in Taiwan.

Institutional Review Board Statement: This study was approved by the Committee on the Ethics of Animal Experiments and was performed according to the Guidelines for Animal Experiments of the China Medical University (#CMUIACUC-2019-284-1; approved July 2019). We have described it in the "Animals".

Informed Consent Statement: Not applicable.

Data Availability Statement: Not applicable.

Acknowledgments: $Stk^{24tm1a(GEMMS)Narl}$ (RMPC13241, MST3-1a/+) was used in this study as previously report [18].

Conflicts of Interest: The authors declare no conflict of interest.

References

1. Kirchner, K.A. Effect of acute potassium infusion on loop segment chloride reabsorption in the rat. *Am. J. Physiol.* **1983**, *244*, F599–F605. [CrossRef]
2. Yang, L.; Xu, S.; Guo, X.; Uchida, S.; Weinstein, A.M.; Wang, T.; Palmer, L.G. Regulation of renal Na transporters in response to dietary K. *Am. J. Physiol. Ren. Physiol.* **2018**, *315*, F1032–F1041. [CrossRef]
3. Sorensen, M.V.; Grossmann, S.; Roesinger, M.; Gresko, N.; Todkar, A.P.; Barmettler, G.; Ziegler, U.; Odermatt, A.; Loffing-Cueni, D.; Loffing, J. Rapid dephosphorylation of the renal sodium chloride cotransporter in response to oral potassium intake in mice. *Kidney Int.* **2013**, *83*, 811–824. [CrossRef] [PubMed]
4. Shoda, W.; Nomura, N.; Ando, F.; Mori, Y.; Mori, T.; Sohara, E.; Rai, T.; Uchida, S. Calcineurin inhibitors block sodium-chloride cotransporter dephosphorylation in response to high potassium intake. *Kidney Int.* **2017**, *91*, 402–411. [CrossRef] [PubMed]
5. Wilson, F.H.; Disse-Nicodeme, S.; Choate, K.A.; Ishikawa, K.; Nelson-Williams, C.; Desitter, I.; Gunel, M.; Milford, D.V.; Lipkin, G.W.; Achard, J.M.; et al. Human hypertension caused by mutations in WNK kinases. *Science* **2001**, *293*, 1107–1112. [CrossRef] [PubMed]
6. Chen, J.C.; Lo, Y.F.; Lin, Y.W.; Lin, S.H.; Huang, C.L.; Cheng, C.J. WNK4 kinase is a physiological intracellular chloride sensor. *Proc. Natl. Acad. Sci. USA* **2019**, *116*, 4502–4507. [CrossRef] [PubMed]
7. Shekarabi, M.; Zhang, J.; Khanna, A.R.; Ellison, D.H.; Delpire, E.; Kahle, K.T. WNK Kinase Signaling in Ion Homeostasis and Human Disease. *Cell Metab.* **2017**, *25*, 285–299. [CrossRef] [PubMed]
8. Terker, A.S.; Zhang, C.; Erspamer, K.J.; Gamba, G.; Yang, C.-L.; Ellison, D.H. Unique chloride-sensing properties of WNK4 permit the distal nephron to modulate potassium homeostasis. *Kidney Int.* **2016**, *89*, 127–134. [CrossRef] [PubMed]
9. Wei, K.-Y.; Gritter, M.; Vogt, L.; de Borst, M.H.; Rotmans, J.I.; Hoorn, E.J. Dietary potassium and the kidney: Lifesaving physiology. *Clin. Kidney J.* **2020**, *13*, 952–968. [CrossRef]
10. Terker, A.S.; Castañeda-Bueno, M.; Ferdaus, M.Z.; Cornelius, R.J.; Erspamer, K.J.; Su, X.T.; Miller, L.N.; McCormick, J.A.; Wang, W.H.; Gamba, G.; et al. With no lysine kinase 4 modulates sodium potassium 2 chloride cotransporter activity in vivo. *Am. J. Physiol. Ren. Physiol.* **2018**, *315*, F781–F790. [CrossRef]
11. Yang, S.S.; Lo, Y.F.; Wu, C.C.; Lin, S.W.; Yeh, C.J.; Chu, P.; Sytwu, H.K.; Uchida, S.; Sasaki, S.; Lin, S.H. SPAK-knockout mice manifest Gitelman syndrome and impaired vasoconstriction. *J. Am. Soc. Nephrol.* **2010**, *21*, 1868–1877. [CrossRef] [PubMed]
12. Lin, S.H.; Yu, I.S.; Jiang, S.T.; Lin, S.W.; Chu, P.; Chen, A.; Sytwu, H.K.; Sohara, E.; Uchida, S.; Sasaki, S.; et al. Impaired phosphorylation of Na(+)-K(+)-2Cl(-) cotransporter by oxidative stress-responsive kinase-1 deficiency manifests hypotension and Bartter-like syndrome. *Proc. Natl. Acad. Sci. USA* **2011**, *108*, 17538–17543. [CrossRef] [PubMed]
13. Rafiqi, F.H.; Zuber, A.M.; Glover, M.; Richardson, C.; Fleming, S.; Jovanovic, S.; Jovanovic, A.; O'Shaughnessy, K.M.; Alessi, D.R. Role of the WNK-activated SPAK kinase in regulating blood pressure. *Embo Mol. Med.* **2010**, *2*, 63–75. [CrossRef] [PubMed]
14. Richardson, C.; Sakamoto, K.; de los Heros, P.; Deak, M.; Campbell, D.G.; Prescott, A.R.; Alessi, D.R. Regulation of the NKCC2 ion cotransporter by SPAK-OSR1-dependent and -independent pathways. *J. Cell Sci.* **2011**, *124*, 789–800. [CrossRef]
15. Kleta, R.; Bockenhauer, D. Salt-Losing Tubulopathies in Children: What's New, What's Controversial? *J. Am. Soc. Nephrol.* **2018**, *29*, 727–739. [CrossRef] [PubMed]
16. Bhalla, V.; Hallows, K.R. Mechanisms of ENaC regulation and clinical implications. *J. Am. Soc. Nephrol.* **2008**, *19*, 1845–1854. [CrossRef] [PubMed]

17. Zhang, C.; Wang, L.; Su, X.T.; Zhang, J.; Lin, D.H.; Wang, W.H. ENaC and ROMK activity are inhibited in the DCT2/CNT of TgWnk4(PHAII) mice. *Am. J. Physiol. Ren. Physiol.* **2017**, *312*, F682–F688. [CrossRef]
18. Lu, T.J.; Kan, W.C.; Yang, S.S.; Jiang, S.T.; Wu, S.N.; Ling, P.; Bao, B.Y.; Lin, C.Y.; Yang, Z.Y.; Weng, Y.P.; et al. MST3 is involved in ENaC-mediated hypertension. *Am. J. Physiol. Ren. Physiol.* **2019**, *317*, F30–F42. [CrossRef]
19. Lu, T.-J.; Chan, C.-H.; Ling, P.; Chao, Y.-M.; Bao, B.-Y.; Chiang, C.-Y.; Lee, T.-H.; Weng, Y.-P.; Kan, W.-C.; Lu, T.-L. MST3 (mammalian Ste20-like protein kinase 3), a novel gene involved in ion homeostasis and renal regulation of blood pressure in spontaneous hypertensive rats. *Int. Urol. Nephrol.* **2018**, *50*, 2299–2307. [CrossRef]
20. Rengarajan, S.; Lee, D.H.; Oh, Y.T.; Delpire, E.; Youn, J.H.; McDonough, A.A. Increasing plasma [K+] by intravenous potassium infusion reduces NCC phosphorylation and drives kaliuresis and natriuresis. *Am. J. Physiol. Ren. Physiol.* **2014**, *306*, F1059–F1068. [CrossRef]
21. He, G.; Wang, H.R.; Huang, S.K.; Huang, C.L. Intersectin links WNK kinases to endocytosis of ROMK1. *J. Clin. Investig.* **2007**, *117*, 1078–1087. [CrossRef] [PubMed]
22. Zhuang, J.; Zhang, X.; Wang, D.; Li, J.; Zhou, B.; Shi, Z.; Gu, D.; Denson, D.D.; Eaton, D.C.; Cai, H. WNK4 kinase inhibits Maxi K channel activity by a kinase-dependent mechanism. *Am. J. Physiol. Ren. Physiol.* **2011**, *301*, F410–F419. [CrossRef] [PubMed]
23. Ares, G.R.; Caceres, P.S.; Ortiz, P.A. Molecular regulation of NKCC2 in the thick ascending limb. *Am. J. Physiol. Ren. Physiol.* **2011**, *301*, F1143–F1159. [CrossRef] [PubMed]
24. Palmer, L.G.; Frindt, G. Aldosterone and potassium secretion by the cortical collecting duct. *Kidney Int.* **2000**, *57*, 1324–1328. [CrossRef] [PubMed]
25. Palmer, B.F.; Clegg, D.J. Physiology and pathophysiology of potassium homeostasis. *Adv. Physiol. Educ.* **2016**, *40*, 480–490. [CrossRef] [PubMed]
26. Grimm, P.R.; Sansom, S.C. BK channels and a new form of hypertension. *Kidney Int.* **2010**, *78*, 956–962. [CrossRef] [PubMed]
27. Rieg, T.; Vallon, V.; Sausbier, M.; Sausbier, U.; Kaissling, B.; Ruth, P.; Osswald, H. The role of the BK channel in potassium homeostasis and flow-induced renal potassium excretion. *Kidney Int.* **2007**, *72*, 566–573. [CrossRef]
28. Shibata, S.; Zhang, J.; Puthumana, J.; Stone, K.L.; Lifton, R.P. Kelch-like 3 and Cullin 3 regulate electrolyte homeostasis via ubiquitination and degradation of WNK4. *Proc. Natl. Acad. Sci. USA* **2013**, *110*, 7838–7843. [CrossRef] [PubMed]
29. Castañeda-Bueno, M.; Arroyo, J.P.; Zhang, J.; Puthumana, J.; Yarborough, O.; Shibata, S.; Rojas-Vega, L.; Gamba, G.; Rinehart, J.; Lifton, R.P. Phosphorylation by PKC and PKA regulate the kinase activity and downstream signaling of WNK4. *Proc. Natl. Acad. Sci. USA* **2017**, *114*, E879–E886. [CrossRef] [PubMed]
30. Lin, D.-H.; Yue, P.; Rinehart, J.; Sun, P.; Wang, Z.; Lifton, R.; Wang, W.-H. Protein phosphatase 1 modulates the inhibitory effect of With-no-Lysine kinase 4 on ROMK channels. *Am. J. Physiol. Ren. Physiol.* **2012**, *303*, F110–F119. [CrossRef] [PubMed]
31. Penton, D.; Czogalla, J.; Wengi, A.; Himmerkus, N.; Loffing-Cueni, D.; Carrel, M.; Rajaram, R.D.; Staub, O.; Bleich, M.; Schweda, F.; et al. Extracellular K(+) rapidly controls NaCl cotransporter phosphorylation in the native distal convoluted tubule by Cl(-) -dependent and independent mechanisms. *J. Physiol.* **2016**, *594*, 6319–6331. [CrossRef] [PubMed]
32. Kan, W.-C.; Lu, T.-L.; Ling, P.; Lee, T.-H.; Cho, C.-Y.; Huang, C.-Y.F.; Jeng, W.-Y.; Weng, Y.-P.; Chiang, C.-Y.; Wu, J.B.; et al. Pervanadate induces Mammalian Ste20 Kinase 3 (MST3) tyrosine phosphorylation but not activation. *J. Inorg. Biochem.* **2016**, *160*, 33–39. [CrossRef] [PubMed]
33. Lu, T.J.; Lai, W.Y.; Huang, C.Y.; Hsieh, W.J.; Yu, J.S.; Hsieh, Y.J.; Chang, W.T.; Leu, T.H.; Chang, W.C.; Chuang, W.J.; et al. Inhibition of cell migration by autophosphorylated mammalian sterile 20-like kinase 3 (MST3) involves paxillin and protein-tyrosine phosphatase-PEST. *J. Biol. Chem.* **2006**, *281*, 38405–38417. [CrossRef] [PubMed]
34. Lu, T.J.; Huang, C.Y.; Yuan, C.J.; Lee, Y.C.; Leu, T.H.; Chang, W.C.; Lu, T.L.; Jeng, W.Y.; Lai, M.D. Zinc ion acts as a cofactor for serine/threonine kinase MST3 and has a distinct role in autophosphorylation of MST3. *J. Inorg. Biochem.* **2005**, *99*, 1306–1313. [CrossRef] [PubMed]

International Journal of
Molecular Sciences

MDPI

Review

Sodium Intake and Heart Failure

Yash Patel [1] **and Jacob Joseph** [2,3,*]

[1] Lifespan Cardiovascular Institute, Warren Alpert Medical School at Brown University, Providence, RI 02914, USA; dryashpatel21@gmail.com
[2] Department of Medicine, Veterans Affairs Boston Healthcare System, Boston, MA 02132, USA
[3] Department of Medicine, Brigham and Women's Hospital, Harvard Medical School, Boston, MA 02115, USA
* Correspondence: jjoseph16@partners.org; Tel.: +1-857-203-6841

Received: 3 November 2020; Accepted: 10 December 2020; Published: 13 December 2020

Abstract: Sodium is an essential mineral and nutrient used in dietary practices across the world and is important to maintain proper blood volume and blood pressure. A high sodium diet is associated with increased expression of β—myosin heavy chain, decreased expression of α/β—myosin heavy chain, increased myocyte enhancer factor 2/nuclear factor of activated T cell transcriptional activity, and increased salt-inducible kinase 1 expression, which leads to alteration in myocardial mechanical performance. A high sodium diet is also associated with alterations in various proteins responsible for calcium homeostasis and myocardial contractility. Excessive sodium intake is associated with the development of a variety of comorbidities including hypertension, chronic kidney disease, stroke, and cardiovascular diseases. While the American College of Cardiology/American Heart Association/Heart Failure Society of America guidelines recommend limiting sodium intake to both prevent and manage heart failure, the evidence behind such recommendations is unclear. Our review article highlights evidence and underlying mechanisms favoring and contradicting limiting sodium intake in heart failure.

Keywords: sodium; salt; heart failure; ambulatory heart failure; epidemiological studies

---

1. Salt and Sodium

Salt is an ionic compound made up of cation and anion. Edible salt consists of 40% sodium and 60% chloride by weight. Salt was historically used as a preservative since bacteria cannot flourish in the presence of high salt concentrations. Human cells require approximately 0.5 g/day of sodium to maintain vital functions. Most food preservatives have high sodium content and are major causes of increased dietary intake of sodium. The average sodium intake in most Americans is 3.4 g/day or 1.5 teaspoons of salt, which is greater than the physiological requirement for the human body. High sodium or salt intake can lead to chronic comorbidities including hypertension, heart failure (HF), chronic kidney disease, stroke, cardiovascular diseases, and increase mortality. Hence, current guidelines recommend restricting sodium consumption to 2–3 g/day [1].

HF is a major burden of morbidity and mortality on the health care system and is classified into two major groups, heart failure with reduced ejection fraction (HFrEF) and heart failure with preserved ejection fraction (HFpEF). Treatment of HFrEF involves both pharmacologic and non-pharmacologic strategies, while mainly heart rate and blood pressure control strategies are used in HFpEF since multiple clinical trials have not shown significant benefits of pharmacologic therapy [2]. Sodium restriction has historically been taught in textbooks as a cornerstone of the management of HF patients. However, data on this management strategy are controversial. In addition, the adherence to following a low sodium diet is challenging, especially after a recent hospitalization, as shown by Riegel et al. [3]. Before we vigorously start educating HF patients to limit sodium intake in their diet, we need to understand the evidence behind such recommendations. In this paper, we review evidence relating sodium to HF, pathophysiological mechanisms of increased sodium intake, and the relation of sodium intake to HF outcomes.

2. Guideline Recommendations for Sodium Intake

A low sodium diet is recommended in most national and international guidelines, as described in Table 1, with the intent of promoting health and preventing and managing comorbidities including HF.

Table 1. Guideline recommendations for sodium restriction in the general population.

Year, Name of Guideline	Sodium Restriction
2010, Dietary Guidelines for Americans [4]	<2.3 g/d in all adults <1.5 g/d in adults aged more than 50 years who are African American or with hypertension, diabetes, or chronic kidney disease
2013, World Health Organization [5]	<2 g/d in all adults
2020, American Heart Association [6]	<1.5 g/d in all adults
2010, Heart Failure Society of America [1]	2–3 g/d in all heart failure patients<2 g/d in patients with moderate to severe heart failure
2019, American Diabetic Association [7]	<2.3 g/d in patients with diabetes<1.5 g/d in patients with diabetes and hypertension
2016, European Society of Cardiology [8]	<5 g/d in all adults
2017, Canadian Cardiovascular Society [9]	<2 g/d in all adults
2015–2020 Dietary Guidelines for Americans [10]	2.3 g/d in all adults
2012, The Kidney disease: Improving Global Outcomes (KDIGO) [11]	<2 g/d in all patients with chronic disease not on dialysis

3. Low Sodium Intake and Prevention or Management of HF

3.1. Evidence in Favor of Low Sodium Intake in Prevention or Management of HF

Systemic hypertension is one of the main risk factors for the development of HF. The lifetime risk of HF decreases with adequate treatment of blood pressure. Data from meta-analysis suggest a dose–response relationship between salt intake and increased blood pressure [12]. In a pooled analysis from four large prospective studies involving 133,118 patients, higher sodium intake was associated with increased risk of cardiovascular events and death compared with moderate sodium intake in hypertensive populations over a median of 4.2 years [13]. Systemic hypertension, if untreated, is a major risk factor for development of left ventricular hypertrophy. In the hypertensive patient population, diastolic dysfunction, left ventricular hypertrophy, and arterial stiffness are associated with urinary sodium excretion, and limiting sodium intake is associated with regression of left ventricular hypertrophy [14–17]. The proposed mechanism of regression of left ventricular hypertrophy with sodium restriction is improved large-arterial stiffness and microvascular endothelial dysfunction [18,19]. Sodium restriction is appropriate in patients with stage A (at risk for HF) and B (asymptomatic) HF due to its effect on lowering blood pressure, the incidence of hypertension, left ventricular hypertrophy, cardiovascular disease, and even incidence of HF [17,20–24]. However, there is insufficient evidence for such recommendation for stage C (with prior or current symptoms) and D (refractory) HF [25]. The Dietary Approaches to Stop Hypertension (DASH) diet, which emphasizes limiting sodium intake, has been shown to be associated with a lower incidence of HF in a prospective observational study of 36,019 participants in the Swedish Mammography Cohort over a course of seven years [26].

3.2. Pathogenic Mechanisms for Beneficial Effect of Low Sodium Intake in Management of HF

Figure 1 shows potential mechanisms of benefit with low sodium intake in patients with HF. A low sodium diet is shown to be associated with decreased pulmonary artery and capillary wedge pressures in patients with New York Heart Association (NYHA) Class III to IV heart failure [27]. Previous studies have shown that HF patients have systemic inflammation characterized by increased levels of tumor necrosis factor *(TNF)-alpha*, interleukin *(IL)-1B* and *IL-6*, chemokine (monocytes chemoattractant protein-1 and IL-8), as well as enhanced expression of adhesion molecules. Moderate sodium restriction (up to 2.8 g/d) was associated with reduced values of neurohormonal (B-type natriuretic peptide (BNP), aldosterone, plasma renin activity) and cytokine levels (*TNF-alpha, IL-6*) and increased levels of anti-inflammatory cytokine (*IL-10*) over 12 months of follow up compared to low sodium restriction (up to 1.8 g/d) [28]. A recent review of the effects of low dietary sodium intake in patients with HF revealed that 2.6–3 g/d of dietary sodium restriction is effective for decreased BNP, renin, and aldosterone plasma levels [29]. Similarly, low sodium intake in the DASH diet is associated with low systolic and diastolic blood pressure, arterial stiffness, and markers of oxidative stress including urinary F2-isiprostane levels in HFpEF patients [30]. Adherence to the DASH diet was shown to be associated with improvement in arterial compliance, improved exercise capacity, and quality of life in patients with stage C HF [31].

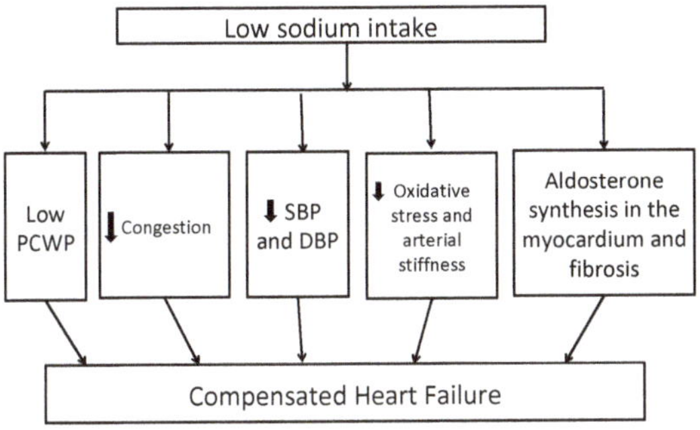

Figure 1. Potential mechanisms linking dietary sodium restriction to better heart failure outcomes DBP—diastolic blood pressure, PCWP—pulmonary capillary wedge pressure, SBP—systolic blood pressure. Abbreviations: DBP, diastolic blood pressure; SBP, systolic blood pressure; PCWP, pulmonary capillary wedge pressure.

4. Low Sodium Intake and Worsening of HF

4.1. Evidence Against Low Sodium Intake in HF

In a randomized clinical trial, Aliti et al. studied the effect of the intervention of <2 g/d of salt intake in patients admitted with acute decompensated HFrEF with EF ≤ 45% on HF clinical congestion score compared to a control group with >2 g/d of salt intake [32]. On 30 days follow-up, there were no differences between the groups in the number of hospital readmissions and length of stay, though the patients in the intervention group had significantly more congestion than the control group ($p = 0.02$) [32]. Similarly, Velloso et al. did not see any significant difference in time needed for resolution of HF symptoms in adult patients admitted to the hospital with acute illness due to underlying chronic HF between the intervention group with <2 g/d salt intake and the control group with more than 2 g/d salt intake [33]. In a large Italian study in patients admitted with HF, patients assigned to low sodium intake (1.84 g/d) compared to moderate sodium intake (2.76 g/d), had reduced diuresis, more HF readmissions, poorer renal function, and a trend towards increased mortality [34]. Subjects in this study did not receive optimal neurohormonal blockade and received strict fluid restriction of 1 L/d and had high diuretic doses (up to 100 to 1000 mg of furosemide) without adjustment of clinical status. A recent pilot study done to see the effects of three-months of 1.5 g versus 3.0 g daily sodium intake in patients with HFrEF showed that both dietary interventions reduced urinary sodium without adverse quality of life improvements [35].

In animal models, sodium restriction in early stages of HF was seen to be associated with early aldosterone activation compared to normal or excess sodium intake [36]. These findings suggest that sodium restriction in early stages of HF should be avoided to prevent neuroendocrine disease progression. The data on sodium and fluid restriction in HFpEF patients are limited. A randomized clinical trial to see the effect of a diet with sodium and fluid restriction compared to an unrestricted diet in patients admitted with acute decompensated HFpEF showed that aggressive sodium and fluid restriction does not decrease readmission and mortality rate, and that it impairs the patient's food intake without any significant neurohormonal effect [37]. A recent systematic review by Mahtani et al. in 2018 including nine randomized control trials that enrolled a total of 479 patients from a total of 2655 retrieved references, revealed no robust high-quality evidence of the effects of sodium restriction in patients with HF [38]. There was a trend in improvement of HF functional class symptoms in outpatient studies with reduced sodium intake, but no effects were observed on all-cause mortality, hospitalization, or length of stay [38]. Similarly, a recent randomized trial of 44 patients hospitalized for acute decompensated HF showed that a normal sodium diet (7 g/d), when compared to a low sodium diet (3 g/d) is associated with similar degrees of decongestion with lower neurohormonal activation during acute HF treatment [39].

4.2. Potential Mechanism for Adverse Impact of Low Sodium Intake in HF

Figure 2 shows the potential mechanism for decompensated HF with low sodium intake. In short, HF is characterized by activation of the sympathetic system and renin–angiotensin–aldosterone system (RAAS) activation due to decreased renal perfusion leading to sodium and water reabsorption from renal tubules [40,41]. A sodium-restricted diet in HF patients has been shown to be associated with activation of antidiuretic and anti-natriuretic systems [42]. A recent Cochrane review of 185 clinical studies randomizing persons to low- vs. high-sodium diet revealed that in plasma or serum, there was a statistically significant increase in renin, aldosterone, noradrenaline, adrenaline, cholesterol, and triglyceride levels in groups with low sodium intake as compared to groups with high sodium intake [43]. These increases in hormones can lead to further development of congestive symptoms. Vascular congestion in HF activates pro-oxidant and pro-inflammatory genes in endothelial cells, which contributes to cardiorenal dysfunction [44–46]. Reduced sodium intake can lower blood pressure, which in turn can increase the heart rate and thereby negate the effects of beta-blockers. This was shown in a recent meta-analysis of 63 studies, although the effect was marginal with a heart rate increase of as little as 2.4% [47]. Reverse causation could also explain the observed association of lower sodium intake and outcomes. Higher-risk individuals with HF might consume less sodium due to their underlying illness but still have higher risks of adverse events.

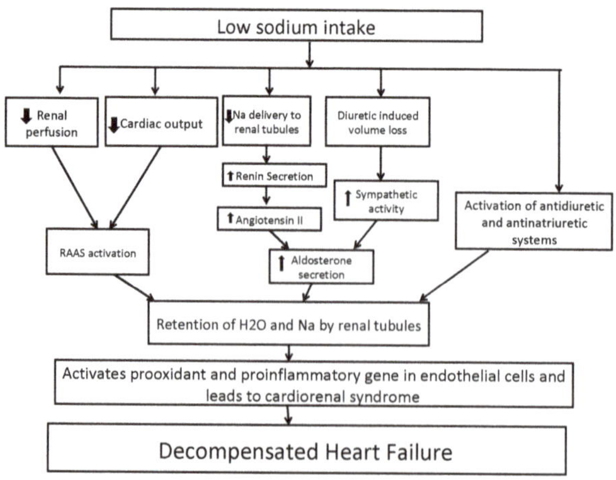

Figure 2. Potential mechanisms whereby dietary sodium restriction may worsen heart failure. Abbreviations: Na, sodium; RAAS, renin–angiotensin–aldosterone system.

5. Potential Molecular Mechanism of Salt Diet and Heart Failure

The myosin heavy chain (*MHC*) protein is formed of α and β filaments. Changes in the proportion of these protein filaments are associated with cardiac mechanical performance. A high sodium diet is associated with an increase in cardiac expression of *β-MHC* and a decrease in the *α/β-MHC* ratio [48]. A low sodium diet was seen to be associated with increased *α/β-MHC* ratio, which in turn improves myocardial mechanical performance [48]. Similar effects of a high sodium diet were seen to be associated with myocyte enhancer factor (*MEF*) 2/nuclear factor of activated T cell (*NFAT*) transcriptional activity, and thereby increasing the expression of *MHC* genes [49]. Systemic hypertension can lead to a shift in the isoform distribution towards overexpression of the *β-MHC* gene with simultaneous downregulation of the *α-MHC* gene [50–52]. A high salt diet is associated with an increase in salt-inducible kinase 1 expression, which mediates the activation of *MEF2/NFAT* and genes associated with left ventricular hypertrophy [49].

There are five main proteins that are involved with calcium homeostasis and myocardial contractility—L-type Ca^{2+} channel (*LTCC*), phospholamban (*PLB*), *SERCA2a*, Na^{+}/Ca^{2+} exchanger (*NCX*), and ryanodine receptors (*RYR*). A high sodium diet is also associated with reduced expression of both *PLB* and *NCX*. Ca^{2+} handling is important to maintain myocardial performance. The *LTCC* plays an important role in action potential during systole. Once Ca^{2+} enters the myocardial cell, it activates *RYR*, which in turn triggers Ca^{2+} release from the sarcoplasmic reticulum. This increase in Ca^{2+} release is responsible for the activation of myocardial contraction during systole. During diastole, the opposite mechanism happens; Ca^{2+} is pumped back from the cytosol to the sarcoplasmic reticulum by *SERCA2a* and sarcolemmal *NCX-1*, which mediates regulation of Ca^{2+} and Na^{+} exchange and thereby maintains excitation–contraction coupling. Altered Ca^{2+} handing is an important pathophysiological mechanism by which preclinical HF develops. Salt restriction has been shown to be associated with decreased *LTCC* protein levels in the left ventricle, increased *PLB* expression, and reduced *NCX* levels. Combined, these mechanisms together decreases sarcoplasmic reticulum Ca^{2+} overload by having an inhibitory effect on *SRCA2a* activity, and thereby is associated with a decrease in the contractility index [53–55].

6. Sodium Intake and Ambulatory Heart Failure

Low-sodium diet recommendations not only apply to hospitalized patients but also to ambulatory patients to prevent acute worsening of symptoms. However, the evidence behind these recommendations is not conclusive. Alvelos et al. reported that in patients with chronic HFrEF with Ejection Fraction (EF) ≤40%, sodium restriction was not associated with improvement in NYHA functional class during 15-day follow-up [42]. Colin-Ramirez et al. in 2004 showed that in patients with HFrEF or HFpEF, 2.0–2.4 g/d of sodium restriction was associated with an improvement in NYHA functional class and less reported signs of HF on 6-months follow up [56]. However, Colin-Ramirez et al. in 2015 showed no significant difference in NYHA functional class between the intervention group with sodium restriction of 1.5 g/d in patients and the control group of moderate sodium intake of 2.4 g/d in patients with HFrEF and HFpEF who are on optimal medical therapy during 6-months follow up [57]. In a study by Philipson et al., sodium and fluid restriction of 2.3 g/d and 1500 mL/d respectively were associated with lower NYHA functional class and symptoms of edema in patients with a history of HF in NYHA classes II and IV over a 12-week follow-up [58]. Hummel et al. reported that 30-day readmissions were lower in the group with sodium restriction of 1.5 g/d in patients with a history of hypertension and recent admission or acute decompensated HF who are followed by discharge into the community [59]. However, they reported that the Kansas City Cardiomyopathy Questionnaire clinical summary score was not different between the two groups over 12 weeks of follow-up [59]. Amongst 123 ambulatory HFrEF patients from two outpatient HF clinics over a median follow-up of three years, higher sodium tertile was associated with a 39% increased risk for all-cause hospitalization and a 3.5-fold increase in risk for mortality [60]. A recent propensity-matched analysis from the HF Adherence and Retention Trial showed that sodium restriction to <2.5 g/d in NYHA class II/III HF patients is associated with a 72% higher risk of death or HF hospitalization compared to a higher sodium intake of >2.5 g/d, especially in patients not receiving therapy with renin–angiotensin antagonists with a hazard ratio of 5.23 [61]. However, sodium intake was determined from a food-frequency questionnaire, which is subject to recall bias.

7. Sodium Intake in Selected Patient Populations

Recent meta-analyses of randomized control trials of treatment of hypertension reveal that the older population, non-white population, and only study groups with blood pressure in the highest 25th percentile show a clinically significant drop in blood pressure with a low sodium diet [62,63]. The Prospective Urban Rural Epidemiology study data showed that an increase in dietary sodium intake is associated with worse cardiovascular morbidity and mortality in a population with high basal sodium intake [64]. A dietary sodium restriction in such a population should be efficacious. Moreover, dietary sodium restriction was not efficacious in a population with low basal serum intake [64]. Amongst The National Health and Nutrition Examination Survey I participants over an average of 19 years of follow-up, a higher intake of dietary sodium was shown to be a strong independent risk factor for HF in overweight men and women with a body mass index of ≥25 kg/m^2 [24]. Such effect was not seen amongst adult U.S. men and women with a body mass index <25 kg/m^2. It also appears that sodium restriction is more beneficial for patients with advanced heart failure symptoms. Amongst 302 patients with HF, greater than 3 g/d dietary sodium intake was found to be associated with a hazard ratio of 2.54 (95% CI 1.10–5.84) for cardiac event-free survival in patients with NYHA III/IV HF symptoms compared to a hazard ratio of 0.44 (95% CI 0.20–0.97) in patients with NYHA I/II HF symptoms [65]. These data suggest that sodium restriction should be applied in only such a targeted population to obtain a substantial benefit. A study by Dolanski et al. examined the association of cognitive decline and low-sodium dietary adherence in 339 HF patients [66]. Interestingly, cognitive decline was not associated with low sodium intake; higher socioeconomic status and higher body mass index was associated with higher sodium intake. Similarly, Creber et al. studied the predictors of high sodium excretion in patients with previously or currently symptomatic HF amongst 280 community-dwelling adults [67]. They found that concomitant obesity and diabetes, and intact instead of deprived cognitive function, were associated with higher odds of sodium excretion. Similarly, sodium consumption was evaluated in 305 outpatients with HFrEF after receiving education to follow a <2 g sodium diet [68]. The authors found that sodium consumption exceeded recommended amounts in men and those with higher body mass indexes. These findings narrate the importance of addressing such demographic discrepancies to target in clinical trials to evaluate clinical outcomes with sodium restriction.

8. Serum Sodium Values and HF

Research has shown that low serum sodium value (hyponatremia) is seen in about 20% of hospitalized patients with acute HF [69]. Serum sodium concentration is closely regulated by water homeostasis, which in turn is regulated by thirst, arginine vasopressin, and kidney function [70]. Hyponatremia can be caused by excessive water retention from neurohormonal activation as well as by negative sodium balance from loop diuretics and with a low sodium intake diet [39]. Serum sodium values can be used to prognosticate outcomes in both HFrEF and HFpEF. Low serum sodium is a risk factor for poor long-term outcomes in acute HF, regardless of ejection fraction [71]. The Organize Program to Initiate Lifesaving Treatment in Hospitalized Patients with Heart Failure registry (OPTIMIZE-HF) involving 48,612 patients recruited from 259 hospitals revealed that each 3 mmol/L drop in serum sodium values below 140 mmol/L in hospitalized patients is associated with a 19.5% increased risk of in-hospital mortality, 10% increased risk of mortality on follow-up, and 8% increase risk of death or rehospitalization on follow-up [69]. A meta-analysis of HF patients showed that low serum sodium values are associated with an increased risk of mortality [72]. We have previously shown in a national Veterans Affairs database study of 25,540 HFpEF patients that a J-shaped relationship is observed between serum sodium levels and a higher risk of number of days of HF hospitalizations and all-cause hospitalizations per year [73]. Such a relationship exists with baseline measurements of serum sodium levels at the time of diagnosis of HF as well as during longitudinal follow-up. Among 50,932 HFpEF patients with a median follow-up of 2.9 years, a J-shaped relationship was seen between serum sodium values and all-cause mortality, HF hospitalizations, and all-cause hospitalizations [74]. These data are further supported by the fact that the improvement of hyponatremia in HF patients is associated with long-term clinical outcomes [75].

9. Future Directions

There are multiple clinical trials that aim to examine if sodium restriction in HF patients is associated with improved clinical outcomes. The Study of Dietary Intervention under 100 MMOL in Heart Failure (SODIUM-HF) is an open-label, multicenter, international, randomized controlled trial in ambulatory patients with chronic HF and aims to assess the effects of dietary sodium restriction on clinical outcomes [76]. The Geriatric out of Hospital Randomized Meal Trial in Heart Failure (GOURMET-HF) is a multicenter, randomized, single-blind, controlled trial of 3-months duration to see the effect of sodium restriction/DASH diet in older patients after discharge from acute decompensated HF admission [59].

10. Our Recommendations

There are likely many potential reasons for conflicting evidence regarding the benefit/harm of sodium restriction. These include heterogeneity of HF patient population studied, lack of uniformity in limiting the amount of sodium restriction per day, unclear data on associated use of fluid restriction, and simultaneous usage of diuretics and neurohormonal blockade agents. Given there is clear evidence of the benefit of limiting sodium intake to prevent various comorbidities leading to HF, we recommend limiting sodium intake in those who are at risk to develop comorbidities to prevent the onset of heart failure. In patients with HF, we recommend to continue limiting sodium intake to prevent morbidity associated with HF. We also recommend avoiding too much limitation in sodium intake as this has been associated with worse outcomes in HF patients.

11. Conclusions

The data supporting the restriction of dietary sodium intake in heart failure patients are unclear. While there appears to be a trend in reducing HF symptoms amongst patients using dietary sodium restriction, there appears to be no effect or slightly higher risk in mortality compared to no sodium restriction. A randomized control trial is hence needed to address this important clinical question.

Author Contributions: Y.P., data extraction and writing original draft; J.J., editing the draft; Y.P. and J.J., responsible for final edits of the draft. All authors have read and agreed to the published version of the manuscript.

Funding: This research received no external funding.

Conflicts of Interest: The authors declare no conflict of interest.

Abbreviations

HF	Heart failure
HFrEF	Heart failure with reduced ejection fraction
HFpEF	Heart failure with preserved ejection fraction
DASH	Dietary Approaches to Stop Hypertension
NYHA	New York Heart Association
TNF	Tumor necrosis factor
IL	Interleukin
BNP	Brain natriuretic factor
RAAS	Renin angiotensin aldosterone system
EF-OPTIMIZE-HF	Ejection Fraction Organize Program to Initiate Lifesaving Treatment in Hospitalized Patients with Heart Failure registry
SODIUM-HF	Study of Dietary Intervention Under 100 MMOL in Heart Failure
GOURMET-HF	Geriatric Out of Hospital Randomized Meal Trial in Heart Failure

References

1. Heart Failure Society of America; Lindenfeld, J.; Albert, N.M.; Boehmer, J.P.; Collins, S.P.; Ezekowitz, J.A.; Givertz, M.M.; Katz, S.D.; Klapholz, M.; Moser, D.K.; et al. HFSA 2010 Comprehensive Heart Failure Practice Guideline. *J. Card. Fail.* **2010**, *16*, e1–e194. [CrossRef] [PubMed]
2. Yancy, C.W.; Jessup, M.; Bozkurt, B.; Butler, J.; Casey, D.E., Jr.; Colvin, M.M.; Drazner, M.H.; Filippatos, G.S.; Fonarow, G.C.; Givertz, M.M.; et al. 2017 ACC/AHA/HFSA Focused Update of the 2013 ACCF/AHA Guideline for the Management of Heart Failure: A Report of the American College of Cardiology/American Heart Association Task Force on Clinical Practice Guidelines and the Heart Failure Society of America. *Circulation* **2017**, *136*, e137–e161. [CrossRef] [PubMed]
3. Riegel, B.; Lee, S.; Hill, J.; Daus, M.; Baah, F.O.; Wald, J.W.; Knafl, G.J. Patterns of adherence to diuretics, dietary sodium and fluid intake recommendations in adults with heart failure. *Heart Lung* **2019**, *48*, 179–185. [CrossRef] [PubMed]
4. 2010 Dietary Guidelines for Americans. Available online: https://health.gov/sites/default/files/2020-01/DietaryGuidelines2010.pdf (accessed on 3 December 2020).
5. Sodium Intake for Adults and Children. Available online: https://www.who.int/nutrition/publications/guidelines/sodium_intake_printversion.pdf (accessed on 3 December 2020).
6. Shaking the Salt Habit to Lower High Blood Pressure. Available online: https://www.heart.org/en/health-topics/high-blood-pressure/changes-you-can-make-to-manage-high-blood-pressure/shaking-the-salt-habit-to-lower-high-blood-pressure-:~{}:text=The%20American%20Heart%20Association%20recommends,blood%20pressure%20and%20heart%20health (accessed on 3 December 2020).
7. Evert, A.B.; Dennison, M.; Gardner, C.D.; Garvey, W.T.; Lau, K.H.K.; MacLeod, J.; Mitri, J.; Pereira, R.F.; Rawlings, K.; Robinson, S.; et al. Nutrition Therapy for Adults With Diabetes or Prediabetes: A Consensus Report. *Diabetes Care* **2019**, *42*, 731–754. [CrossRef]
8. Piepoli, M.F.; Hoes, A.W.; Agewall, S.; Albus, C.; Brotons, C.; Catapano, A.L.; Cooney, M.T.; Corra, U.; Cosyns, B.; Deaton, C.; et al. 2016 European Guidelines on cardiovascular disease prevention in clinical practice: The Sixth Joint Task Force of the European Society of Cardiology and Other Societies on Cardiovascular Disease Prevention in Clinical Practice (constituted by representatives of 10 societies and by invited experts)Developed with the special contribution of the European Association for Cardiovascular Prevention & Rehabilitation (EACPR). *Eur. Heart J.* **2016**, *37*, 2315–2381. [CrossRef]
9. Ezekowitz, J.A.; O'Meara, E.; McDonald, M.A.; Abrams, H.; Chan, M.; Ducharme, A.; Giannetti, N.; Grzeslo, A.; Hamilton, P.G.; Heckman, G.A.; et al. 2017 Comprehensive Update of the Canadian Cardiovascular Society Guidelines for the Management of Heart Failure. *Can. J. Cardiol.* **2017**, *33*, 1342–1433. [CrossRef]
10. Cut down on Sodium. Available online: https://health.gov/sites/default/files/2019-10/DGA_Cut-Down-On-Sodium.pdf (accessed on 3 December 2020).
11. KDIGO 2012 Clinical Practice Guideline for the Evaluation and Management of Chronic Kidney Disease. Available online: https://kdigo.org/wp-content/uploads/2017/02/KDIGO_2012_CKD_GL.pdf (accessed on 3 December 2020).
12. He, F.J.; Li, J.; Macgregor, G.A. Effect of longer term modest salt reduction on blood pressure: Cochrane systematic review and meta-analysis of randomised trials. *BMJ* **2013**, *346*, f1325. [CrossRef]
13. Mente, A.; O'Donnell, M.; Rangarajan, S.; Dagenais, G.; Lear, S.; McQueen, M.; Diaz, R.; Avezum, A.; Lopez-Jaramillo, P.; Lanas, F.; et al. Associations of urinary sodium excretion with cardiovascular events in individuals with and without hypertension: A pooled analysis of data from four studies. *Lancet* **2016**, *388*, 465–475. [CrossRef]
14. Schmieder, R.E.; Messerli, F.H.; Garavaglia, G.E.; Nunez, B.D. Dietary salt intake. A determinant of cardiac involvement in essential hypertension. *Circulation* **1988**, *78*, 951–956. [CrossRef]
15. Safar, M.E.; Temmar, M.; Kakou, A.; Lacolley, P.; Thornton, S.N. Sodium intake and vascular stiffness in hypertension. *Hypertension* **2009**, *54*, 203–209. [CrossRef]
16. Langenfeld, M.R.; Schobel, H.; Veelken, R.; Weihprecht, H.; Schmieder, R.E. Impact of dietary sodium intake on left ventricular diastolic filling in early essential hypertension. *Eur. Heart J.* **1998**, *19*, 951–958. [CrossRef] [PubMed]

17. Jula, A.M.; Karanko, H.M. Effects on left ventricular hypertrophy of long-term nonpharmacological treatment with sodium restriction in mild-to-moderate essential hypertension. *Circulation* **1994**, *89*, 1023–1031. [CrossRef] [PubMed]
18. Jablonski, K.L.; Racine, M.L.; Geolfos, C.J.; Gates, P.E.; Chonchol, M.; McQueen, M.B.; Seals, D.R. Dietary sodium restriction reverses vascular endothelial dysfunction in middle-aged/older adults with moderately elevated systolic blood pressure. *J. Am. Coll. Cardiol.* **2013**, *61*, 335–343. [CrossRef] [PubMed]
19. Salvi, P.; Giannattasio, C.; Parati, G. High sodium intake and arterial stiffness. *J. Hypertens.* **2018**, *36*, 754–758. [CrossRef]
20. He, F.J.; Li, J.; Macgregor, G.A. Effect of longer-term modest salt reduction on blood pressure. *Cochrane Database Syst. Rev.* **2013**, CD004937. [CrossRef]
21. The Trials of Hypertension Prevention Collaborative Research Group. Effects of weight loss and sodium reduction intervention on blood pressure and hypertension incidence in overweight people with high-normal blood pressure. The Trials of Hypertension Prevention, phase II. *Arch. Intern. Med.* **1997**, *157*, 657–667. [CrossRef]
22. Cook, N.R.; Cutler, J.A.; Obarzanek, E.; Buring, J.E.; Rexrode, K.M.; Kumanyika, S.K.; Appel, L.J.; Whelton, P.K. Long term effects of dietary sodium reduction on cardiovascular disease outcomes: Observational follow-up of the trials of hypertension prevention (TOHP). *BMJ* **2007**, *334*, 885–888. [CrossRef]
23. Strazzullo, P.; D'Elia, L.; Kandala, N.B.; Cappuccio, F.P. Salt intake, stroke, and cardiovascular disease: Meta-analysis of prospective studies. *BMJ* **2009**, *339*, b4567. [CrossRef]
24. He, J.; Ogden, L.G.; Bazzano, L.A.; Vupputuri, S.; Loria, C.; Whelton, P.K. Dietary sodium intake and incidence of congestive heart failure in overweight US men and women: First National Health and Nutrition Examination Survey Epidemiologic Follow-up Study. *Arch. Intern. Med.* **2002**, *162*, 1619–1624. [CrossRef]
25. Gupta, D.; Georgiopoulou, V.V.; Kalogeropoulos, A.P.; Dunbar, S.B.; Reilly, C.M.; Sands, J.M.; Fonarow, G.C.; Jessup, M.; Gheorghiade, M.; Yancy, C.; et al. Dietary sodium intake in heart failure. *Circulation* **2012**, *126*, 479–485. [CrossRef]
26. Levitan, E.B.; Wolk, A.; Mittleman, M.A. Consistency with the DASH diet and incidence of heart failure. *Arch. Intern. Med.* **2009**, *169*, 851–857. [CrossRef] [PubMed]
27. Cody, R.J.; Covit, A.B.; Schaer, G.L.; Laragh, J.H.; Sealey, J.E.; Feldschuh, J. Sodium and water balance in chronic congestive heart failure. *J. Clin. Investig.* **1986**, *77*, 1441–1452. [CrossRef] [PubMed]
28. Parrinello, G.; Di Pasquale, P.; Licata, G.; Torres, D.; Giammanco, M.; Fasullo, S.; Mezzero, M.; Paterna, S. Long-term effects of dietary sodium intake on cytokines and neurohormonal activation in patients with recently compensated congestive heart failure. *J. Card. Fail.* **2009**, *15*, 864–873. [CrossRef] [PubMed]
29. Lee, Y.W.; Huang, L.H.; Ku, C.H. Use of dietary sodium intervention effect on neurohormonal and fluid overload in heart failure patients: Review of select research based literature. *Appl. Nurs. Res.* **2018**, *42*, 17–21. [CrossRef]
30. Hummel, S.L.; Seymour, E.M.; Brook, R.D.; Kolias, T.J.; Sheth, S.S.; Rosenblum, H.R.; Wells, J.M.; Weder, A.B. Low-sodium dietary approaches to stop hypertension diet reduces blood pressure, arterial stiffness, and oxidative stress in hypertensive heart failure with preserved ejection fraction. *Hypertension* **2012**, *60*, 1200–1206. [CrossRef]
31. Vidal, E.R.; Cabrini, R.; Figueroa, M.A.; Bazzi, L.R.; Parisier, H.; Sanchez Zinny, J. Nodular goiter in young patients. Frequency of thyroid cancer. *Rev. Argent. Cir.* **1965**, *8*, 99–104.
32. Aliti, G.B.; Rabelo, E.R.; Clausell, N.; Rohde, L.E.; Biolo, A.; Beck-da-Silva, L. Aggressive fluid and sodium restriction in acute decompensated heart failure: A randomized clinical trial. *JAMA Intern. Med.* **2013**, *173*, 1058–1064. [CrossRef]
33. Velloso, L.G.; Alonso, R.R.; Ciscato, C.M.; Barretto, A.C.; Bellotti, G.; Pileggi, F. Diet with usual quantity of salt in hospital treatment of congestive heart insufficiency. *Arq. Bras. Cardiol.* **1991**, *57*, 465–468.
34. Paterna, S.; Fasullo, S.; Parrinello, G.; Cannizzaro, S.; Basile, I.; Vitrano, G.; Terrazzino, G.; Maringhini, G.; Ganci, F.; Scalzo, S.; et al. Short-term effects of hypertonic saline solution in acute heart failure and long-term effects of a moderate sodium restriction in patients with compensated heart failure with New York Heart Association class III (Class C) (SMAC-HF Study). *Am. J. Med. Sci.* **2011**, *342*, 27–37. [CrossRef]

35. Kalogeropoulos, A.; Papadimitriou, L.; Georgiopoulou, V.V.; Dunbar, S.B.; Skopicki, H.; Butler, J. Low-Versus Moderate-Sodium Diet in Patients With Recent Hospitalization for Heart Failure: The PROHIBIT (Prevent Adverse Outcomes in Heart Failure by Limiting Sodium) Pilot Study. *Circ. Heart Fail.* **2020**, *13*, e006389. [CrossRef]
36. Miller, W.L.; Borgeson, D.D.; Grantham, J.A.; Luchner, A.; Redfield, M.M.; Burnett, J.C., Jr. Dietary sodium modulation of aldosterone activation and renal function during the progression of experimental heart failure. *Eur. J. Heart Fail.* **2015**, *17*, 144–150. [CrossRef]
37. Machado d'Almeida, K.S.; Rabelo-Silva, E.R.; Souza, G.C.; Trojahn, M.M.; Santin Barilli, S.L.; Aliti, G.; Rohde, L.E.; Biolo, A.; Beck-da-Silva, L. Aggressive fluid and sodium restriction in decompensated heart failure with preserved ejection fraction: Results from a randomized clinical trial. *Nutrition* **2018**, *54*, 111–117. [CrossRef] [PubMed]
38. Mahtani, K.R.; Heneghan, C.; Onakpoya, I.; Tierney, S.; Aronson, J.K.; Roberts, N.; Hobbs, F.D.R.; Nunan, D. Reduced Salt Intake for Heart Failure: A Systematic Review. *JAMA Intern. Med.* **2018**, *178*, 1693–1700. [CrossRef] [PubMed]
39. Fabricio, C.G.; Tanaka, D.M.; Souza Gentil, J.R.; Ferreira Amato, C.A.; Marques, F.; Schwartzmann, P.V.; Schmidt, A.; Simoes, M.V. A normal sodium diet preserves serum sodium levels during treatment of acute decompensated heart failure: A prospective, blind and randomized trial. *Clin. Nutr. ESPEN* **2019**, *32*, 145–152. [CrossRef] [PubMed]
40. Selektor, Y.; Weber, K.T. The salt-avid state of congestive heart failure revisited. *Am. J. Med. Sci.* **2008**, *335*, 209–218. [CrossRef]
41. Schrier, R.W. Body fluid volume regulation in health and disease: A unifying hypothesis. *Ann. Intern. Med.* **1990**, *113*, 155–159. [CrossRef] [PubMed]
42. Alvelos, M.; Ferreira, A.; Bettencourt, P.; Serrao, P.; Pestana, M.; Cerqueira-Gomes, M.; Soares-Da-Silva, P. The effect of dietary sodium restriction on neurohumoral activity and renal dopaminergic response in patients with heart failure. *Eur. J. Heart Fail.* **2004**, *6*, 593–599. [CrossRef]
43. Graudal, N.A.; Hubeck-Graudal, T.; Jurgens, G. Effects of low sodium diet versus high sodium diet on blood pressure, renin, aldosterone, catecholamines, cholesterol, and triglyceride. *Cochrane Database Syst. Rev.* **2011**, CD004022. [CrossRef]
44. Colombo, P.C.; Banchs, J.E.; Celaj, S.; Talreja, A.; Lachmann, J.; Malla, S.; DuBois, N.B.; Ashton, A.W.; Latif, F.; Jorde, U.P.; et al. Endothelial cell activation in patients with decompensated heart failure. *Circulation* **2005**, *111*, 58–62. [CrossRef]
45. Damman, K.; van Deursen, V.M.; Navis, G.; Voors, A.A.; van Veldhuisen, D.J.; Hillege, H.L. Increased central venous pressure is associated with impaired renal function and mortality in a broad spectrum of patients with cardiovascular disease. *J. Am. Coll. Cardiol.* **2009**, *53*, 582–588. [CrossRef]
46. Mullens, W.; Abrahams, Z.; Francis, G.S.; Sokos, G.; Taylor, D.O.; Starling, R.C.; Young, J.B.; Tang, W.H.W. Importance of venous congestion for worsening of renal function in advanced decompensated heart failure. *J. Am. Coll. Cardiol.* **2009**, *53*, 589–596. [CrossRef] [PubMed]
47. Graudal, N.A.; Hubeck-Graudal, T.; Jurgens, G. Reduced Dietary Sodium Intake Increases Heart Rate. A Meta-Analysis of 63 Randomized Controlled Trials Including 72 Study Populations. *Front. Physiol.* **2016**, *7*, 111. [CrossRef] [PubMed]
48. Berger, R.C.M.; Benetti, A.; Girardi, A.C.C.; Forechi, L.; de Oliveira, R.M.; Vassallo, P.F.; Mill, J.G. Influence of Long-Term Salt Diets on Cardiac Ca2+ Handling and Contractility Proteins in Hypertensive Rats. *Am. J. Hypertens.* **2018**, *31*, 726–734. [CrossRef] [PubMed]
49. Popov, S.; Venetsanou, K.; Chedrese, P.J.; Pinto, V.; Takemori, H.; Franco-Cereceda, A.; Eriksson, P.; Mochizuki, N.; Soares-da-Silva, P.; Bertorello, A.M. Increases in intracellular sodium activate transcription and gene expression via the salt-inducible kinase 1 network in an atrial myocyte cell line. *Am. J. Physiol.-Heart Circ. Physiol.* **2012**, *303*, H57–H65. [CrossRef]
50. Gupta, M.; Gupta, M.P. Cardiac hypertrophy: Old concepts, new perspectives. *Mol. Cell. Biochem.* **1997**, *176*, 273–279. [CrossRef]
51. Lowes, B.D.; Minobe, W.; Abraham, W.T.; Rizeq, M.N.; Bohlmeyer, T.J.; Quaife, R.A.; Roden, R.L.; Dutcher, D.L.; Robertson, A.D.; Voelkel, N.F.; et al. Changes in gene expression in the intact human heart. Downregulation of alpha-myosin heavy chain in hypertrophied, failing ventricular myocardium. *J. Clin. Investig.* **1997**, *100*, 2315–2324. [CrossRef]

52. Ling, Q.; Chen, T.H.; Guo, Z.G. Inhibition of beta-myosin heavy chain gene expression in pressure overload rat heart by losartan and captopril. *Zhongguo Yao Li Xue Bao* **1997**, *18*, 63–66.
53. Cantilina, T.; Sagara, Y.; Inesi, G.; Jones, L.R. Comparative studies of cardiac and skeletal sarcoplasmic reticulum ATPases. Effect of a phospholamban antibody on enzyme activation by Ca2+. *J. Biol. Chem.* **1993**, *268*, 17018–17025.
54. Kadambi, V.J.; Ponniah, S.; Harrer, J.M.; Hoit, B.D.; Dorn, G.W., 2nd; Walsh, R.A.; Kranias, E.G. Cardiac-specific overexpression of phospholamban alters calcium kinetics and resultant cardiomyocyte mechanics in transgenic mice. *J. Clin. Investig.* **1996**, *97*, 533–539. [CrossRef]
55. Masaki, H.; Sako, H.; Kadambi, V.J.; Sato, Y.; Kranias, E.G.; Yatani, A. Overexpression of phospholamban alters inactivation kinetics of L-type Ca2+ channel currents in mouse atrial myocytes. *J. Mol. Cell. Cardiol.* **1998**, *30*, 317–325. [CrossRef]
56. Colin Ramirez, E.; Castillo Martinez, L.; Orea Tejeda, A.; Rebollar Gonzalez, V.; Narvaez David, R.; Asensio Lafuente, E. Effects of a nutritional intervention on body composition, clinical status, and quality of life in patients with heart failure. *Nutrition* **2004**, *20*, 890–895. [CrossRef] [PubMed]
57. Colin-Ramirez, E.; McAlister, F.A.; Zheng, Y.; Sharma, S.; Armstrong, P.W.; Ezekowitz, J.A. The long-term effects of dietary sodium restriction on clinical outcomes in patients with heart failure. The SODIUM-HF (Study of Dietary Intervention Under 100 mmol in Heart Failure): A pilot study. *Am. Heart J.* **2015**, *169*, 274–281. [CrossRef] [PubMed]
58. Philipson, H.; Ekman, I.; Forslund, H.B.; Swedberg, K.; Schaufelberger, M. Salt and fluid restriction is effective in patients with chronic heart failure. *Eur. J. Heart Fail.* **2013**, *15*, 1304–1310. [CrossRef] [PubMed]
59. Wessler, J.D.; Maurer, M.S.; Hummel, S.L. Evaluating the safety and efficacy of sodium-restricted/Dietary Approaches to Stop Hypertension diet after acute decompensated heart failure hospitalization: Design and rationale for the Geriatric OUt of hospital Randomized MEal Trial in Heart Failure (GOURMET-HF). *Am. Heart J.* **2015**, *169*, 342–348. [CrossRef]
60. Arcand, J.; Ivanov, J.; Sasson, A.; Floras, V.; Al-Hesayen, A.; Azevedo, E.R.; Mak, S.; Allard, J.P.; Newton, G.E. A high-sodium diet is associated with acute decompensated heart failure in ambulatory heart failure patients: A prospective follow-up study. *Am. J. Clin. Nutr.* **2011**, *93*, 332–337. [CrossRef]
61. Doukky, R.; Avery, E.; Mangla, A.; Collado, F.M.; Ibrahim, Z.; Poulin, M.F.; Richardson, D.; Powell, L.H. Impact of Dietary Sodium Restriction on Heart Failure Outcomes. *JACC Heart Fail.* **2016**, *4*, 24–35. [CrossRef]
62. Graudal, N.; Hubeck-Graudal, T.; Jurgens, G.; Taylor, R.S. Dose-response relation between dietary sodium and blood pressure: A meta-regression analysis of 133 randomized controlled trials. *Am. J. Clin. Nutr.* **2019**, *109*, 1273–1278. [CrossRef]
63. Huang, L.; Trieu, K.; Yoshimura, S.; Neal, B.; Woodward, M.; Campbell, N.R.C.; Li, Q.; Lackland, D.T.; Leung, A.A.; Anderson, C.A.M.; et al. Effect of dose and duration of reduction in dietary sodium on blood pressure levels: Systematic review and meta-analysis of randomised trials. *BMJ* **2020**, *368*, m315. [CrossRef]
64. Mente, A.; O'Donnell, M.; Rangarajan, S.; McQueen, M.; Dagenais, G.; Wielgosz, A.; Lear, S.; Ah, S.T.L.; Wei, L.; Diaz, R.; et al. Urinary sodium excretion, blood pressure, cardiovascular disease, and mortality: A community-level prospective epidemiological cohort study. *Lancet* **2018**, *392*, 496–506. [CrossRef]
65. Lennie, T.A.; Song, E.K.; Wu, J.R.; Chung, M.L.; Dunbar, S.B.; Pressler, S.J.; Moser, D.K. Three gram sodium intake is associated with longer event-free survival only in patients with advanced heart failure. *J. Card. Fail.* **2011**, *17*, 325–330. [CrossRef]
66. Dolansky, M.A.; Schaefer, J.T.; Hawkins, M.A.; Gunstad, J.; Basuray, A.; Redle, J.D.; Fang, J.C.; Josephson, R.A.; Moore, S.M.; Hughes, J.W. The association between cognitive function and objective adherence to dietary sodium guidelines in patients with heart failure. *Patient Prefer. Adherence* **2016**, *10*, 233–241. [CrossRef] [PubMed]
67. Masterson Creber, R.; Topaz, M.; Lennie, T.A.; Lee, C.S.; Puzantian, H.; Riegel, B. Identifying predictors of high sodium excretion in patients with heart failure: A mixed effect analysis of longitudinal data. *Eur. J. Cardiovasc. Nurs.* **2014**, *13*, 549–558. [CrossRef] [PubMed]
68. Basuray, A.; Dolansky, M.; Josephson, R.; Sattar, A.; Grady, E.M.; Vehovec, A.; Gunstad, J.; Redle, J.; Fang, J.; Hughes, J.W. Dietary sodium adherence is poor in chronic heart failure patients. *J. Card. Fail.* **2015**, *21*, 323–329. [CrossRef] [PubMed]

69. Gheorghiade, M.; Abraham, W.T.; Albert, N.M.; Gattis Stough, W.; Greenberg, B.H.; O'Connor, C.M.; She, L.; Yancy, C.W.; Young, J.; Fonarow, G.C.; et al. Relationship between admission serum sodium concentration and clinical outcomes in patients hospitalized for heart failure: An analysis from the OPTIMIZE-HF registry. *Eur. Heart J.* **2007**, *28*, 980–988. [CrossRef] [PubMed]
70. Kokko, J.P. The role of the renal concentrating mechanisms in the regulation of serum sodium concentration. *Am. J. Med.* **1977**, *62*, 165–169. [CrossRef]
71. Vicent, L.; Alvarez-Garcia, J.; Gonzalez-Juanatey, J.R.; Rivera, M.; Segovia, J.; Worner, F.; Bover, R.; Pascual-Figal, D.; Vazquez, R.; Cinca, J.; et al. Prognostic impact of hyponatremia and hypernatremia at admission and discharge in heart failure patients with preserved, mid-range, and reduced ejection fraction. *Intern. Med. J.* **2020**. [CrossRef] [PubMed]
72. Rusinaru, D.; Tribouilloy, C.; Berry, C.; Richards, A.M.; Whalley, G.A.; Earle, N.; Poppe, K.K.; Guazzi, M.; Macin, S.M.; Komajda, M.; et al. Relationship of serum sodium concentration to mortality in a wide spectrum of heart failure patients with preserved and with reduced ejection fraction: An individual patient data meta-analysis(dagger): Meta-Analysis Global Group in Chronic heart failure (MAGGIC). *Eur. J. Heart Fail.* **2012**, *14*, 1139–1146. [CrossRef]
73. Patel, Y.R.; Kurgansky, K.E.; Imran, T.F.; Orkaby, A.R.; McLean, R.R.; Ho, Y.L.; Cho, K.; Gaziano, J.M.; Djousse, L.; Gagnon, D.R.; et al. Prognostic Significance of Baseline Serum Sodium in Heart Failure With Preserved Ejection Fraction. *J. Am. Heart Assoc.* **2018**, *7*, e007529. [CrossRef]
74. Imran, T.F.; Kurgansky, K.E.; Patel, Y.R.; Orkaby, A.R.; McLean, R.R.; Ho, Y.L.; Cho, K.; Gaziano, J.M.; Djousse, L.; Gagnon, D.R.; et al. Serial sodium values and adverse outcomes in heart failure with preserved ejection fraction. *Int. J. Cardiol.* **2019**, *290*, 119–124. [CrossRef]
75. Wang, J.; Zhou, W.; Yin, X. Improvement of hyponatremia is associated with lower mortality risk in patients with acute decompensated heart failure: A meta-analysis of cohort studies. *Heart Fail. Rev.* **2019**, *24*, 209–217. [CrossRef]
76. Colin-Ramirez, E.; Arcand, J.; Woo, E.; Brum, M.; Morgan, K.; Christopher, W.; Velazquez, L.; Sharifzad, A.; Feeney, S.; Ezekowitz, J.A. Design and Region-Specific Adaptation of the Dietary Intervention Used in the SODIUM-HF Trial: A Multicentre Study. *CJC Open* **2020**, *2*, 8–14. [CrossRef] [PubMed]

International Journal of
Molecular Sciences

Review

Sodium Intake and Chronic Kidney Disease

Silvio Borrelli [1,*,†], Michele Provenzano [2,†], Ida Gagliardi [2], Michael Ashour [2], Maria Elena Liberti [1], Luca De Nicola [1], Giuseppe Conte [1], Carlo Garofalo [1] and Michele Andreucci [2]

1 Nephrology Unit, Advanced Surgical and Medical Sciences Department of University of Campania "Luigi Vanvitelli", Piazza Miraglia, 80137 Naples, Italy; m.elenaliberti@libero.it (M.E.L.); luca.denicola@unicampania.it (L.D.N.); giuseppe.conte@unicampania.it (G.C.); carlo.garofalo@hotmail.it (C.G.)

2 Nephrology Unit, Department of Health Sciences, *"Magna Grecia"* University, 88100 Catanzaro, Italy; michiprov@hotmail.it (M.P.); ida_88@libero.it (I.G.); ashourmichael@yahoo.com (M.A.); andreucci@unicz.it (M.A.)

* Correspondence: dott.silvioborrelli@gmail.com; Tel.: +39-081-2549405

† These authors contributed equally to this work.

Received: 30 May 2020; Accepted: 1 July 2020; Published: 3 July 2020

Abstract: In Chronic Kidney Disease (CKD) patients, elevated blood pressure (BP) is a frequent finding and is traditionally considered a direct consequence of their sodium sensitivity. Indeed, sodium and fluid retention, causing hypervolemia, leads to the development of hypertension in CKD. On the other hand, in non-dialysis CKD patients, salt restriction reduces BP levels and enhances anti-proteinuric effect of renin–angiotensin–aldosterone system inhibitors in non-dialysis CKD patients. However, studies on the long-term effect of low salt diet (LSD) on cardio-renal prognosis showed controversial findings. The negative results might be the consequence of measurement bias (spot urine and/or single measurement), reverse epidemiology, as well as poor adherence to diet. In end-stage kidney disease (ESKD), dialysis remains the only effective means to remove dietary sodium intake. The mismatch between intake and removal of sodium leads to fluid overload, hypertension and left ventricular hypertrophy, therefore worsening the prognosis of ESKD patients. This imposes the implementation of a LSD in these patients, irrespective of the lack of trials proving the efficacy of this measure in these patients. LSD is, therefore, a rational and basic tool to correct fluid overload and hypertension in all CKD stages. The implementation of LSD should be personalized, similarly to diuretic treatment, keeping into account the volume status and true burden of hypertension evaluated by ambulatory BP monitoring.

Keywords: salt intake; sodium; hypertension; cardiovascular risk; mortality; prognosis

1. Introduction

Sodium is not only considered an important mineral in maintaining the balance of body fluid, but it has also played an important role in the history of the world for its economical, religious, and symbolic importance. The concept that salt is a beneficial substance was so ingrained that although the earlier studies on the relationship between low sodium intake and reduction of blood pressure (BP) date back to 1948 [1], it was only after nearly forty years that the international community has recognized the role of salt intake in the pathophysiology of hypertension [2]. According to the World Health Organization, the restriction of sodium intake to less than 2.3 g/day of sodium corresponding to 5.8 g of salt (or 100 mmol) is one of the most cost-effective measures to improve public health [3]. Cumulating evidence highlights that higher sodium consumption contributes to higher BP [4], thus increasing the risk of cardiovascular disease (CVD) [5,6]. However, recent studies have raised some concerns about the real benefit of a low salt diet in the healthy general population [7–10]. In particular, in a large cohort study in over 100,000 patients from 18 countries the role of higher salt consumption was associated with increased BP levels [7], and poor CV outcomes [8]. At the same time, it emerged that sodium intake of <3 g forecasted a higher CV risk, drawing a U-shaped mortality curve [8]. Although these findings have also been obtained by other investigators [8–10], these studies are methodologically flawed by reverse causality (e.g., patients eat less salt because they are sicker and/or more malnourished), collinearity (e.g., a low sodium intake may be associated with a low protein-energy intake) and biased methods used to assess individual salt intake (e.g., single spot urine sample) [11].

In Chronic Kidney Disease (CKD) patients, high BP is a frequent finding, which is traditionally considered as a direct consequence of sodium sensitivity. Hence, a low salt diet (LSD) is widely considered a cornerstone in the treatment of hypertension in CKD.

In this review, we address the importance of the kidney in sodium regulation, the relationship of sodium intake with hypertension from earlier CKD stages to end-stage kidney disease (ESKD), and the available evidence on the benefit of salt restriction in non-dialysis CKD and in the ESKD population.

2. Adherence to Low-Salt Diet: Definition and Assessment in CKD Patients

The terms sodium and salt (generally sodium chloride) are used interchangeably, generating confusion about sodium intake. Table 1 illustrates formulas to convert sodium in salt (sodium chloride) and *vice versa*, according to the units of measurement.

Table 1. Formulas to convert sodium in salt (sodium chloride) and vice versa, according to units of measurement.

grams of sodium = mmol of sodium × 0.023
grams of salt = mmol of sodium × 0.058 (or mmol of sodium/17)
grams of sodium = grams of salt × 0.394
grams of salt = grams of sodium × 2.542

The first concern in the evaluation of adherence to LSD is the method used for evaluation of sodium intake. Accordingly, the measurement of sodium excretion by 24 h urine sample collection (UNaV) is considered as the gold standard. However, UNaV may be cumbersome for the patient, and, therefore, estimation from spot urine samples using the Nerbass, Kawasaki, Tanaka, and INTERSALT formulas have been proposed to evaluate sodium intake. The rationale arises from the assumption that spot urine excretion would be proportionate to UNaV corrected for creatinine excretion. However, a cross-sectional study in CKD patients showed that these formulas might provide an inaccurate estimate of sodium intake, irrespective of severity of CKD and use of diuretics [12].

Another issue is the evaluation of salt intake by a single measurement, which is not generally considered sufficient to evaluate an individual's usual salt intake because of the wide day-to-day variability in salt consumption and urinary excretion [13].

Among CKD cohorts, the Chronic Renal Insufficiency Cohort (CRIC) study reported that only about one out of four patients had a sodium intake <100 mmol/24 h, evaluated by three measurements [14]. As reported in Table 2, these findings are consistent with the prevalence of LSD reported in secondary analyses of trials [15–19], and also when CKD patients were regularly followed in nephrology clinics (<25% had a salt intake below 6 g/day) [20].

Table 2. Studies evaluating the effect of urinary sodium excretion (UNaV) on end-stage kidney disease (ESKD) and cardiovascular (CV) outcomes in patients with or without Chronic Kidney Disease (CKD).

Author [ref], Year	Type	Sample Size	Mean eGFR	Method to Assess UNaV	Prevalence LSD	ESKD	CV Outcomes
Torres, V.E. [21], 2017	Post-hoc analysis HALT-PKD trial (Study B)	486	48.6	Multiple 24 h urine sample	n.a.	Averaged UNaV is associated with increased risk for the combined endpoint of death, ESRD or 50% eGFR decline [HR 1.08 (1.01–1.06) per 18 mmol/day]	n.a.
He, J. [14], 2016	Longitudinal prospective CRIC study	3757	43.4	Three 24 h urine sample	27.7% (<116 mmol/day)	Highest quartile of UNaV (>194.6 mmol/day) is associated with higher risk of ESKD [HR: 1.46 (1.09–1.70)]	n.a.
Mills, K.T. [22], 2016	Longitudinal prospective CRIC study	3757	43.4	sodium/creatinine ratio from multiple 24 h urine samples	25.0% (<2894 mg/g)	n.a.	Highest quartile of calibrated UNaV (>4548 mg/g) is associated with higher risk of composite CV endpoints [HR: 1.36 (1.09–1.70)]
Fan, L. [16],2014	Post-hoc analysis MDRD trial	840	32.5	Three or four 24-h urine sample	25.0% (<93 mmol/day)	No association was found between mean baseline UnaV and ESKD [HR 0.99 (95% CI 0.91–1.08)]	n.a.
Smyth, A. [17], 2014	Post-hoc analysis ONTARGET TRANSCEND trials	28,879	68.4	Single fasting urine sample	2.7% (<87 mmol/day)	There was no association between estimated UNaV and risk of renal outcomes (ESKD or 30% eGFR decline)	n.a.
Vegter, S. [15], 2012	Post-hoc analysis of REIN1 and -2 trials	500	43.2	sodium/creatinine ratio from multiple 24 h urine samples	22.2% (<100 mmol/day)	Unadjusted analysis showed association between UNaV and renal outcome, which disappears after adjustment for proteinuria	n.a.
Lambers Heerspink, H.J. [18], 2012	Post-hoc analysis of RENAAL and IDNT trials	1177	44.0	sodium/creatinine ratio from multiple 24 h urine samples	33.3% (<121 mmol/day)	In the group of patients treated with ARBs, thelowest UNaV tertiles of were associated with improved renal outcome [HR: 0.57 (0.39–0.84)]	In the group of patients treated with ARBs, the lowest UNaV tertiles were associated with improved CV outcome [HR: 0.54 (0.34–0.86)]
Thomas, M.C. [19], 2011	Longitudinal prospective Study	2807	n.a.	a single 24 h urine collection	25% (<102 mmol/day)	In diabetic patients, UnaV was inversely associated with the cumulative incidence of ESRD.	n.a.

Abbreviations: n.a.: not applicable. ARBs: Angiotensin Receptor Blockers.

Novel methods for self-monitoring of salt intake have been developed to improve the adherence to the LSD; these are based on urine chloride strips, given that urinary chloride excretion is very tightly correlated with urinary sodium excretion. The potential benefit of self-monitoring is the ability to immediately achieve an adequate estimate of sodium intake immediately (75.5% sensitivity and 82.6% specificity to correctly classify patients with UNaV >100 mmol/24 h) in order to make proper dietary adjustments aimed at achieving recommended intake [23]. However, any benefit on the achievement of the BP goal with use of chloride strips has still to be proved with use of chloride strips. To answer this question, one randomized clinical trial, the SALUTE-CKD (SALt lowering by Urine sodium self-measurement Trial in Chronic Kidney DiseasE) has advanced to the final stage of development and results are expected in the next few months.

Furthermore, a recent trial performed in 99 patients has evaluated the efficacy of a web-based self-management program for dietary sodium restriction compared with routine care. After 3 months in intervention group a significant reduction of sodium intake (−40 mmol/day) and systolic BP (−8 mmHg) was registered in the intervention group, whereas no significant difference was found in control group. Surprisingly, in the following maintenance phase, no difference in sodium intake was detected between the two groups, due to the inadvertent adoption of the intervention by the control group. Notably, the largest effect was reported in the first 3 months, when participants actively used the web-based self-management program [24].

In ESKD patients, sodium intake can be estimated with a dietary questionnaire, though several factors, such as high dialysate sodium concentration and sodium plasma concentration, can affect thirsty and water intake in these patients, irrespective of their sodium intake [25].

Finally, in ESKD patients, residual kidney function must be carefully evaluated: in this subgroup of patients, dialysis is started with an incremental approach, corresponding to a low dose of dialysis (peritoneal or hemodialysis) integrated into the conservative management [26,27]. In these patients, the assessment of sodium intake by UNaV may be misleading, because of the aliquot of sodium intake removed by dialysis.

3. Hypertension and Salt in CKD

Hypertension and CKD are common chronic noncommunicable diseases strictly inter-related with each other; indeed, elevated BP is not only a frequent complication of CKD [28], but it can also act as the cause of CKD [29]. A recent meta-analysis showed that hypertensive patients have a 75% greater risk than normotensive individuals of development of *de novo* CKD (GFR <60 mL/min/1.73 m^2), estimating a 10% increase of CKD onset for each increase of 10 mmHg of either BP component. Notably, even pre-hypertension (Systolic BP of 120–139 mm Hg and/or Diastolic BP of 80–89 mm Hg) was associated with a 25% higher risk of developing low GFR [29].

Furthermore, the prognostic role of lowering BP assumes greater importance in CKD patients if we bear in mind at least three basic points: (1) higher prevalence of hypertension in CKD than in the general population, which increases progressively from 65% to 95% as GFR falls from 85 to 15 mL/min/1.73 m^2 [29]; (2) hypertension is the main known risk factor for CKD progression and for CV mortality [30]; (3) Hypertension is often resistant to the treatment in CKD patients, resulting in worsening CV prognosis [31,32].

Salt and water retention play a key role for development of hypertension in CKD. In fact, according to the classical model, under normal conditions, high salt intake temporarily increases plasma sodium level, which is soon buffered by movement of water from the intracellular to the extracellular compartment. Thus, increased plasma sodium concentration also stimulates the thirst center, leading to an increase in water intake and secretion of antidiuretic hormone, which restores plasma sodium concentration to a normal level while increasing and maintaining extracellular fluid volume. On the other hand, high salt intake suppresses the renin-angiotensin-aldosterone system (RAAS), which consequently reduces sodium tubular reabsorption, thus contributing to re-establishing sodium and water homeostasis [33].

In CKD patients, external sodium balance is preserved by expansion of the extracellular volume (ECV), which however causes the persistence of high BP levels. Therefore, hypertension in CKD is an early manifestation of ECV expansion and, at the same time, a maladaptive mechanism aimed at limiting ECV expansion that corresponds to approximately 5% to 10% of body weight, generally without peripheral edema, when cardiac and hepatic function is normal and the transcapillary Starling forces are not disrupted [34]. In spite of ECV expansion, RAAS is inappropriately activated in CKD, leading to vasoconstriction and sodium retention, which contribute significantly to the raising of BP levels [35].

As reported in a classic experiment [36], the BP response to sodium load is amplified in CKD patients. In particular, increasing sodium intake was increased from 20 to 120 mmol/day in patients with advanced renal failure, this caused a significant acute increase of BP (+12.2 ± 1.4 mmHg). On the other hand, the same increase in sodium intake in healthy people was not associated with any BP change and, even greater elevation of sodium intake up to 1120 mmol/day, did not produce any effect on BP values. This experiment is the proof of concept of the sodium sensitivity of BP in CKD. Notably, sodium sensitivity may be already detectable in the earlier CKD stages, as reported in a study comparing patients with glomerular disease vs healthy controls, which showed a significant BP reduction in response to lowering salt intake, whereas BP did not change in controls [37].

Moreover, experimental studies showed that high salt intake induces intrarenal production of Angiotensin-II [38], stimulates the synthesis of pro-inflammatory cytokines [39] and increases oxidative stress [40], as well as triggering sympathetic activity [41], whose activation is already increased in CKD, as a result of increased arterial stiffness and/or endothelial dysfunction [42].

4. Alternative Mechanism of Sodium Toxicity

Recent experimental findings suggest that skin could work as a reservoir of sodium, escaping from renal control [43]. In particular, high salt intake might cause sodium accumulation in the skin, which is detected by cells of the Monocytes Phagocytes System (MPS) located in the skin interstitium, which act as osmoreceptors by expression of the tonicity enhancer-binding protein (Ton-EBP). This transcription factor leads to Vascular Endothelial Growth Factor (VEGF) production that increases sodium clearance by the lymphatic network [44,45]. Moreover, high sodium levels in the CKD condition would promote the expression of pro-inflammatory factors, such as Interleukin-6, VEGF, and Monocyte Chemoattractant Protein-1 (MCP-1), via Ton-EBP pathway, leading to local inflammation and vascular proliferation in peritoneal, heart, and vascular tissue [46].

Figure 1 summarizes the potential mechanisms underlying the increase of BP levels and dependent CV risk associated with high salt intake in CKD.

The concept that sodium balance is regulated by additional extra-renal mechanisms was first reported by Herr et al., whose study showed that high salt intake increased total sodium content, whereas total body water and body weight did not change [47]. More recently, a space flight simulation study has reported that in healthy subjects under controlled sodium intake, UNaV changes periodically (every 6 days), independently from BP levels and total body water [48].

The recent availability of ^{23}Na Magnetic Resonance Imaging (MRI) in humans has allowed detection and quantification of sodium storage in the skin [49]. In particular, a higher tissue sodium content was detected in patients affected by hyperaldosteronism. Interestingly, surgical and/or medical correction of hyperaldosteronism was associated with a significant reduction in tissue sodium content; whereas body weight did not change [50]. Recently, in a cross-sectional analysis of 99 CKD patients, skin sodium content was strongly associated with left ventricular mass independently from BP levels and volume status [51]. Finally, sodium stored into the skin is modifiable in CKD patients, as reported by a recent study showing a significant reduction of skin sodium content, after a single hemodialysis session, though the mechanism by which sodium is removed from skin remains still unclear [52].

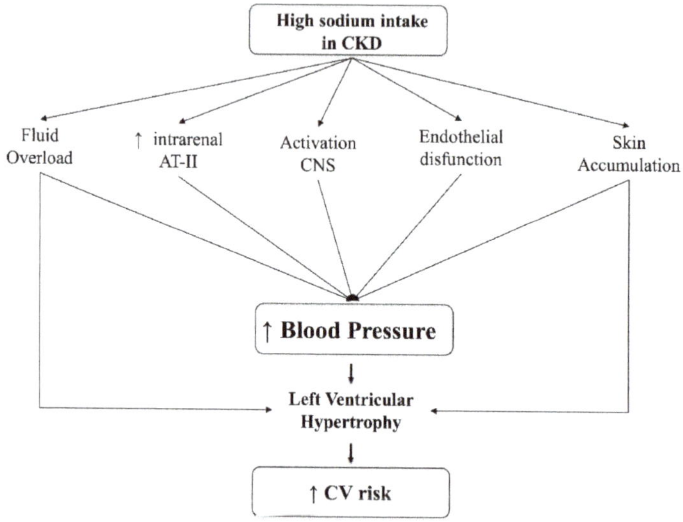

Figure 1. Potential pathogenic mechanisms of hypertension in CKD due to high salt intake. Abbreviations: CKD: Chronic Kidney Disease; AT-II: Angiotensin-II; CNS; Central Nervous System; CV: cardiovascular.

5. Clinical Effects of Low Salt Diet in Non-Dialysis CKD

We have recently completed a metanalysis comparing low versus high salt diet in 738 CKD patients [53]. Analysis included nine trials [54–62]. This meta-analysis showed that a moderate salt restriction of 4.4 g/day (from 179 mEq/day to 104 mEq/day) was associated with a significant lowering of 4.9 mmHg [95% C.I.: 6.8/3.1 mmHg; $p < 0.001$] in systolic BP and of 2.3 mmHg [95% C.I.: 6.8/3.1 mmHg; $p < 0.001$] in diastolic BP measured by traditional method [53]. A similar effect was found in the five out of eleven studies [57,60,61,63,64] evaluating the effect of LSD on Ambulatory BP (ABP). In particular, we found that salt restriction reduces systolic and diastolic ABP of 5.9 mmHg (95% C.I.: 2.3/9.5 mmHg; $p < 0.001$) and 3.0 mmHg (95% C.I.: 1.7/4.7 mmHg; $p < 0.001$), respectively [53].

As regards ABP studies, it is worth mentioning that in CKD cohorts, sodium sensitivity has been associated with a higher prevalence of altered circadian rhythm and nocturnal hypertension [65,66], which are predictors of poor cardio-renal prognosis [67].

Moreover, in seven out of eleven studies [54–59] reporting the effect of salt restriction on proteinuria, pooled analysis showed a significant improvement of 0.4 g/day (95% C.I.: 0.2–0.6 g/day) associated with lower salt intake [53]. These findings are in agreement with a previous meta-analysis reporting that in patients following a lower salt diet, there was an augmented antiproteinuric effect of RAAS blockers [68]. The synergic effect of LSD and RAAS inhibition may be correlated to the finding that high salt intake enhances angiotensin-converting enzyme (ACE) activity in renal tissues, in spite of decreased plasma renin and angiotensinogen concentrations, which could reduce the effect of RAAS blockers in tissues [38].

Although these effects of LSD on BP and proteinuria suggest an improvement of prognosis in CKD patients, few studies [14–19] have evaluated the long-term effect of salt restriction on the cardio-renal outcomes (Table 2).

In the CRIC study, a large observational study carried out in 3757 CKD patients followed for almost seven years, the group of patients with a UnaV of >195 mmol/day was associated with a higher risk of CKD progression [14]. Among participants of this study, 804 composite CV events (575 heart failure, 305 myocardial infarctions, and 148 strokes) occurred during a median of 6.8 years of follow-up, drawing a linear relation between higher sodium intake and higher CV risk [22]. Similarly, a post-hoc analysis of the Reduction of Endpoints in NIDDM with the Angiotensin II Antagonist Losartan (RENAAL) and Irbesartan Diabetic Nephropathy Trial (IDNT) trials in a subgroup of 1177 patients with available 24 h urinary sodium measurements, showed that the beneficial effects of RAAS blockers on renal and cardiovascular outcomes were greater in patients with lower sodium intake [18]. Furthermore, in Autosomal Dominant Polycystic Kidney Disease (ADPKD) patients, fast progressors irrespective of intensive CKD management [69,70], a recent post-hoc analysis of the HALT-PKD trial has shown that a moderate salt restriction reduces CKD progression [21].

On the other hand, other studies have not confirmed these results, finding no association between low salt intake and improvement of the renal prognosis, in CKD patients [15–17]. In particular, secondary analysis of the first and second Ramipril Efficacy in Nephropathy (REIN) trials showed that low salt intake was associated with a lower risk of ESKD, but this association disappeared after adjustment for basal proteinuria [15]. In the longitudinal follow up of the Modification of Diet in Renal Disease (MDRD) Study, no association of single baseline 24 h urinary sodium excretion with kidney failure and a composite outcome of kidney failure or all-cause mortality was found [16]. Similarly, post-hoc analysis of the ongoing telmisartan alone and in combination with ramipril global endpoint trial (ONTARGET) and telmisartan randomized assessment study in ACE intolerant subjects with cardiovascular disease (TRANSCEND) studies trials showed no association between UNaV (though estimated by morning spot urine) and renal endpoints (30% decline of eGFR or ESKD) in patients with or without CKD at baseline [17]. Surprisingly, in diabetic non-CKD patients, UNaV was inversely associated with a cumulative incidence of ESKD, and in fact, patients with the lowest sodium excretion had the highest cumulative incidence of ESKD [19].

Of note, the negative studies are post hoc analyses of clinical trials designed to test the efficacy of RAAS inhibitors rather than of low-sodium intervention, confounding thus a possible association [15–18]. Furthermore, in some of these studies, UNaV was measured by a single 24 h urine [19] or spot urine sample [17]. On the other hand, we cannot exclude that other factors might play a role: a renal hemodynamic response to an acute reduction of sodium intake was impaired by aging, especially when atherosclerotic damage coexists [71]. This may expose patients to acute kidney injury and hypotension [72]. Furthermore, patients with CKD have a higher prevalence of white coat effect [73,74], exposing CKD patients to "inappropriate" antihypertensive treatment, which may potentially cause renal hypoperfusion [75]. Therefore, particular attention must be paid in the management of CKD patients, personalizing salt intake on the basis of "true" hypertensive status measured by ABPM and volemic status, and monitoring the adherence and anti-hypertensive effect LSD over time.

6. Sodium Intake in End-Stage Kidney Disease

In ESKD patients, similarly to early CKD stages (Figure 1), the deleterious effects of high salt intake are mainly related to the fluid overload, resulting in high BP levels, left ventricular hypertrophy, and increased CV mortality [76–80]. Therefore, sodium restriction is a major therapeutic goal in these patients. Indeed, it has been estimated that, in ESKD patients with no residual diuresis, a salt intake of <6 g should cause patients to gain no more than 0.8 kg/day in interdialytic weight.

A recent metanalysis of four trials (3 in HD/1 in PD) showed that ESKD patients with lower salt intake (N = 67) had a significant improvement of both systolic [−8.4 (−12.0; −4,8) mmHg] and diastolic BP [−4.4 (−6.6; −4.2) mmHg] levels compared with the higher salt intake group (N = 64) [81]. Moreover, a post-hoc analysis of the HEMO study revealed that low sodium intake, evaluated by a 24 h food questionnaire, allowed to decrease the need for ultrafiltration, even if it was not associated with pre-dialysis systolic BP levels [82].

Similarly, hypervolemia is prevalent in Peritoneal Dialysis (PD) patients, because of the common mismatch between intake and removal of sodium and fluid [83–85]. In a recent study performed in a cohort of 1054 incident PD patients, overhydration was evident in over 50% of patients starting PD [83]. This finding is relevant because persistence of volume overload heralds a 60% higher mortality risk [84]. Interestingly, recent experimental findings have reported that high sodium intake is related to direct toxicity on the peritoneal membrane, leading to chronic inflammation, fibrosis, and hypervascularization, increasing, in turn, peritoneal permeability [86].

Surprisingly, few studies have addressed the relationship between sodium intake and mortality in ESKD patients (Table 3). In hemodialysis, secondary analysis of HEMO study showed that higher dietary sodium correlated with mortality rate independently from patients' nutritional status [82]. A retrospective study on 305 Chinese PD patients has reported that sodium intake, assessed by a 3-day diet questionnaire, was inversely associated with all-cause and cardiovascular mortality. It is noteworthy that patients with lower sodium intake also had lower serum albumin levels and reduced lean body mass, as well as lower energy and protein intake, when compared with patients with higher sodium intake, suggesting that patients with a lower dietary sodium intake were more malnourished and with reduced appetite. Moreover, the group of patients with highest salt intake had mean sodium intake of 2.5 g/day, which is lower than the mean intake reported in the general population, suggesting a possible measurement bias. This study, moreover, was flawed by methodological issues (small sample size, monocentric, few events, and overfitted cox models), further reducing the generalizability of the results [87].

Table 3. Studies evaluating the effect of urinary sodium excretion (UNaV) on mortality in ESKD patients.

Author [ref], Year	Type	Sample Size	Dietary Sodium Evaluation	Outcomes
Hemodialysis				
McCausland [82], 2012	Post-hoc analysis of HEMO trial	1170	48 h food diary	Higher dietary salt intake is associated with greater mortality.
Peritoneal Dialysis				
Dong [87], 2010	Retrospective analysis	305	3-day dietary records	Higher dietary salt intake is associated with lower mortality (aHR:0.45 (0.23–0.90)

Therefore, salt restriction remains the basic approach to achieve volume control in PD patients, keeping in mind that sodium removal is lower in PD patients treated with cycler (Automated PD, APD), because of greater sodium sieving as compared with Continuous Ambulatory PD (CAPD). In these patients, high salt intake may not be counterbalanced by sodium removal, consequently leading to hypervolemia and hypertension [88].

7. Conclusions

The negative effects of sodium on BP values are amplified in CKD patients, as a result of fluid overload and of direct toxicity on the heart, the vascular system, and kidney. In non-dialysis CKD patients, LSD is beneficial for hypertension control, irrespective of BP levels, to lower proteinuria by enhancing the antiproteinuric effect of RAAS inhibition. Whether these effects can improve cardio-renal prognosis still remains unclear. Nonetheless, salt restriction assumes a greater importance in ESKD because of the common mismatch between intake and removal of sodium, which leads to hypertension, LVH, and higher CV risk. Therefore, reducing salt intake is crucial for hypertensive CKD patients from earlier stages to ESKD. However, it remains insufficiently and/or inadequately applied. More studies are therefore needed to improve adherence to LSD in the long term.

Author Contributions: S.B.: Data curation, Writing - original draft; M.P.: Data curation, Funding acquisition, Writing - original draft; I.G.: Funding acquisition Writing - review & editing; M.A. (Michael Ashour) and M.A. (Michele Andreucci): Funding acquisition Writing - review & editing; M.E.L., L.D.N., C.G. and G.C.: Supervision Writing - review & editing. All authors have read and agreed to the published version of the manuscript.

Funding: This research received no external funding.

Conflicts of Interest: The authors declare no conflict of interest.

References

1. Kempner, W. Some Effects of the Rice Diet Treatment of Kidney Disease and Hypertension. *Bull. N. Y. Acad. Med.* **1946**, *22*, 358–370.
2. Kotchen, T.A.; Cowley AWJr Frohlich, E.D. Salt in health and disease—A delicate balance. *N. Engl. J. Med.* **2013**, *368*, 1229–1237. [CrossRef] [PubMed]
3. World Health Organization. *Guideline: Sodium Intake for Adults and Children*; World Health Organization: Geneva, Switzerland, 2012; pp. 1–46.
4. He, F.J.; Li, J.; Macgregor, G.A. Effect of longer term modest salt reduction on blood pressure: Cochrane systematic review and meta-analysis of randomized trials. *BMJ* **2013**, *346*, f1325. [CrossRef] [PubMed]
5. He, F.J.; MacGregor, G.A. Salt reduction lowers cardiovascular risk: Meta-analysis of outcome trials. *Lancet* **2011**, *378*, 380–382. [CrossRef]
6. Strazzullo, P.; D'Elia, L.; Kandala, N.B.; Cappuccio, F.P. Salt intake, stroke, and cardiovascular disease: Meta-analysis of prospective studies. *BMJ* **2009**, *339*, b4567. [CrossRef]
7. Mente, A.; O'Donnell, M.J.; Rangarajan, S.; McQueen, M.J.; Poirier, P.; Wielgosz, A.; Morrison, H.; Li, W.; Wang, X.; Di, C.; et al. Association of urinary sodium and potassium excretion with blood pressure. *N. Engl. J. Med.* **2014**, *371*, 601–611. [CrossRef]
8. O'Donnell, M.; Mente, A.; Rangarajan, S.; McQueen, M.J.; Wang, X.; Liu, L.; Yan, H.; Lee, S.F.; Mony, P.; Devanath, A.; et al. Urinary sodium and potassium excretion, mortality, and cardiovascular events. *N. Engl. J. Med.* **2014**, *371*, 612–623. [CrossRef]
9. Graudal, N.; Jürgens, G.; Baslund, B.; Alderman, M.H. Compared with usual sodium intake, low- and excessive-sodium diets are associated with increased mortality: A meta-analysis. *Am. J. Hypertens.* **2014**, *27*, 1129–1137. [CrossRef]
10. Stolarz-Skrzypek, K.; Kuznetsova, T.; Thijs, L.; Tikhonoff, V.; Seidlerová, J.; Richart, T.; Jin, Y.; Olszanecka, A.; Malyutina, S.; Casiglia, E.; et al. Fatal and nonfatal outcomes, incidence of hypertension, and blood pressure changes in relation to urinary sodium excretion. *JAMA* **2011**, *305*, 1777–1785. [CrossRef]
11. Whelton, P.K.; Appel, L.J.; Sacco, R.L.; Anderson, C.A.; Antman, E.M.; Campbell, N.; Dunbar, S.B.; Frohlich, E.D.; Hall, J.E.; Jessup, M.; et al. Sodium, blood pressure, and cardiovascular disease: Further evidence supporting the American Heart Association sodium reduction recommendations. *Circulation* **2012**, *126*, 2880–2889. [CrossRef]
12. Dougher, C.E.; Rifkin, D.E.; Anderson, C.A.; Smits, G.; Persky, M.S.; Block, G.A.; Ix, J.H. Spot urine sodium measurements do not accurately estimate dietary sodium intake in chronic kidney disease. *Am. J. Clin. Nutr.* **2016**, *104*, 298–305. [CrossRef] [PubMed]
13. Olde Engberink, R.H.G.; van den Hoek, T.C.; van Noordenne, N.D.; van den Born, B.H.; Peters-Sengers, H.; Vogt, L. Use of a Single Baseline Versus Multiyear 24-Hour Urine Collection for Estimation of Long-Term Sodium Intake and Associated Cardiovascular and Renal Risk. *Circulation* **2017**, *136*, 917–926. [CrossRef] [PubMed]
14. He, J.; Mills, K.T.; Appel, L.J.; Yang, W.; Chen, J.; Lee, B.T.; Rosas, S.E.; Porter, A.; Makos, G.; Weir, M.R.; et al. Urinary Sodium and Potassium Excretion and CKD Progression. *J. Am. Soc. Nephrol.* **2016**, *27*, 1202–1212. [CrossRef] [PubMed]
15. Vegter, S.; Perna, A.; Postma, M.J.; Navis, G.; Remuzzi, G.; Ruggenenti, P. Sodium intake, ACE inhibition, and progression to ESRD. *J. Am. Soc. Nephrol.* **2012**, *23*, 165–173. [CrossRef]
16. Fan, L.; Tighiouart, H.; Levey, A.S.; Beck, G.J.; Sarnak, M.J. Urinary sodium excretion and kidney failure in nondiabetic chronic kidney disease. *Kidney Int.* **2014**, *86*, 582–588. [CrossRef]
17. Smyth, A.; Dunkler, D.; Gao, P.; Teo, K.K.; Yusuf, S.; O'Donnell, M.J.; Mann, J.F.; Clase, C.M. ONTARGET and TRANSCEND investigators. The relationship between estimated sodium and potassium excretion and subsequent renal outcomes. *Kidney Int.* **2014**, *86*, 1205–1212. [CrossRef]
18. Lambers Heerspink, H.J.; Holtkamp, F.A.; Parving, H.H.; Navis, G.J.; Lewis, J.B.; Ritz, E.; de Graeff, P.A.; de Zeeuw, D. Moderation of dietary sodium potentiates the renal and cardiovascular protective effects of angiotensin receptor blockers. *Kidney Int.* **2012**, *82*, 330–337. [CrossRef]
19. Thomas, M.C.; Moran, J.; Forsblom, C.; Harjutsalo, V.; Thorn, L.; Ahola, A.; Wadén, J.; Tolonen, N.; Saraheimo, M.; Gordin, D.; et al. The association between dietary sodium intake, ESRD, and all-cause mortality in patients with type 1 diabetes. *Diabetes Care* **2011**, *34*, 861–866. [CrossRef]

20. De Nicola, L.; Chiodini, P.; Zoccali, C.; Borrelli, S.; Cianciaruso, B.; Di Iorio, B.; Santoro, D.; Giancaspro, V.; Abaterusso, C.; Gallo, C.; et al. Prognosis of CKD patients receiving outpatient nephrology care in Italy. *Clin. J. Am. Soc. Nephrol.* **2011**, *6*, 2421–2428. [CrossRef]
21. Torres, V.E.; Abebe, K.Z.; Schrier, R.W.; Perrone, R.D.; Chapman, A.B.; Yu, A.S.; Braun, W.E.; Steinman, T.I.; Brosnahan, G.; Hogan, M.C.; et al. Dietary salt restriction is beneficial to the management of autosomal dominant polycystic kidney disease. *Kidney Int.* **2017**, *91*, 493–500. [CrossRef]
22. Mills, K.T.; Chen, J.; Yang, W.; Appel, L.J.; Kusek, J.W.; Alper, A.; Delafontaine, P.; Keane, M.G.; Mohler, E.; Ojo, A.; et al. Sodium Excretion and the Risk of Cardiovascular Disease in Patients With Chronic Kidney Disease. *JAMA* **2016**, *315*, 2200–2210. [CrossRef] [PubMed]
23. Panuccio, V.; Pizzini, P.; Parlongo, G.; Caridi, G.; Tripepi, R.; Mafrica, A.; Cutrupi, S.; D'Arrigo, G.; Porto, G.; Garofalo, C.; et al. Urine chloride self-measurement to monitor sodium chloride intake in patients with chronic kidney disease. *Clin. Chem. Lab. Med.* **2019**, *57*, 1162–1168. [CrossRef] [PubMed]
24. Humalda, J.K.; Klaassen, G.; de Vries, H.; Meuleman, Y.; Verschuur, L.C.; Straathof, E.J.M.; Laverman, G.D.; Bos, W.J.W.; van der Boog, P.J.M.; Vermeulen, K.M.; et al. A Self-management Approach for Dietary Sodium Restriction in Patients With CKD: A Randomized Controlled Trial. *Am. J. Kidney Dis.* **2020**, *75*, 847–856. [CrossRef] [PubMed]
25. Lindley, E.J. Reducing sodium intake in hemodialysis patients. *Semin. Dial.* **2009**, *22*, 260–263. [CrossRef]
26. Garofalo, C.; Borrelli, S.; De Stefano, T.; Provenzano, M.; Andreucci, M.; Cabiddu, G.; La Milia, V.; Vizzardi, V.; Sandrini, M.; Cancarini, G.; et al. Incremental dialysis in ESRD: Systematic review and meta-analysis. *J. Nephrol.* **2019**, *32*, 823–836. [CrossRef]
27. Bellizzi, V.; Conte, G.; Borrelli, S.; Cupisti, A.; De Nicola, L.; Di Iorio, B.R.; Cabiddu, G.; Mandreoli, M.; Paoletti, E.; Piccoli, G.B.; et al. Controversial issues in CKD clinical practice: Position statement of the CKD-treatment working group of the Italian Society of Nephrology. *J. Nephrol.* **2017**, *30*, 159–170. [CrossRef]
28. Klag, M.J.; Whelton, P.K.; Randall, B.L.; Neaton, J.D.; Brancati, F.L.; Ford, C.E.; Shulman, N.B.; Stamler, J. Blood pressure and end-stage renal disease in men. *N. Engl. J. Med.* **1996**, *334*, 13–18. [CrossRef]
29. Garofalo, C.; Borrelli, S.; Pacilio, M.; Minutolo, R.; Chiodini, P.; De Nicola, L.; Conte, G. Hypertension and Prehypertension and Prediction of Development of Decreased Estimated GFR in the General Population: A Meta-analysis of Cohort Studies. *Am. J. Kidney Dis.* **2016**, *67*, 89–97. [CrossRef]
30. Chang, A.R.; Lóser, M.; Malhotra, R.; Appel, L.J. Blood Pressure Goals in Patients with CKD: A Review of Evidence and Guidelines. *Clin. J. Am. Soc. Nephrol.* **2019**, *14*, 161–169. [CrossRef]
31. Borrelli, S.; De Nicola, L.; Stanzione, G.; Conte, G.; Minutolo, R. Resistant hypertension in nondialysis chronic kidney disease. *Int. J. Hypertens.* **2013**, *2013*, 929183. [CrossRef]
32. De Nicola, L.; Gabbai, F.B.; Agarwal, R.; Chiodini, P.; Borrelli, S.; Bellizzi, V.; Nappi, F.; Conte, G.; Minutolo, R. Prevalence and prognostic role of resistant hypertension in chronic kidney disease patients. *J. Am. Coll. Cardiol.* **2013**, *61*, 2461–2467. [CrossRef] [PubMed]
33. Guyton, A.C. Kidneys and fluids in pressure regulation. Small volume but large pressure changes. *Hypertension* **1992**, *19* (Suppl. 1), I2. [CrossRef] [PubMed]
34. De Nicola, L.; Minutolo, R.; Bellizzi, V.; Zoccali, C.; Cianciaruso, B.; Andreucci, V.E.; Fuiano, G.; Conte, G.; Investigators of the TArget Blood Pressure LEvels in Chronic Kidney Disease (TABLE in CKD) Study Group. Achievement of target blood pressure levels in chronic kidney disease: A salty question? *Am. J. Kidney Dis.* **2004**, *43*, 782–795. [CrossRef] [PubMed]
35. Laurent, S.; Boutouyrie, P. The structural factor of hypertension: Large and small artery alterations. *Circ. Res.* **2015**, *116*, 1007–1021. [CrossRef] [PubMed]
36. Koomans, H.A.; Roos, J.C.; Dorhout Mees, E.J.; Delawi, I.M. Sodium balance in renal failure. A comparison of patients with normal subjects under extremes of sodium intake. *Hypertension* **1985**, *7*, 714–721. [CrossRef]
37. Cianciaruso, B.; Bellizzi, V.; Minutolo, R.; Colucci, G.; Bisesti, V.; Russo, D.; Conte, G.; De Nicola, L. Renal adaptation to dietary sodium restriction in moderate renal failure resulting from chronic glomerular disease. *J. Am. Soc. Nephrol.* **1996**, *7*, 306–313.
38. Kobori, H.; Nishiyama, A.; Abe, Y.; Navar, L.G. Enhancement of intrarenal angiotensinogen in Dahl salt-sensitive rats on high salt diet. *Hypertension* **2003**, *41*, 592–597. [CrossRef]
39. Ying, W.Z.; Sanders, P.W. Dietary salt modulates renal production of transforming growth factor-beta in rats. *Am. J. Physiol.* **1998**, *274*, F635–F641. [CrossRef]

40. Meng, S.; Roberts, L.J., II; Cason, G.W.; Curry, T.S.; Manning, R.D., Jr. Superoxide dismutase and oxidative stress in Dahl salt-sensitive and -resistant rats. *Am. J. Physiol. Regul. Integr. Comp. Physiol.* **2002**, *283*, R732–R738. [CrossRef]
41. Guild, S.J.; McBryde, F.D.; Malpas, S.C.; Barrett, C.J. High dietary salt and angiotensin II chronically increase renal sympathetic nerve activity: A direct telemetric study. *Hypertension* **2012**, *59*, 614–620. [CrossRef]
42. Chesterton, L.J.; Sigrist, M.K.; Bennett, T.; Taal, M.W.; McIntyre, C.W. Reduced baroreflex sensitivity is associated with increased vascular calcification and arterial stiffness. *Nephrol. Dial. Transpl.* **2005**, *20*, 1140–1147. [CrossRef]
43. Titze, J.; Dahlmann, A.; Lerchl, K.; Kopp, C.; Rakova, N.; Schröder, A.; Luft, F.C. Spooky sodium balance. *Kidney Int.* **2014**, *85*, 759–767. [CrossRef]
44. Machnik, A.; Neuhofer, W.; Jantsch, J.; Dahlmann, A.; Tammela, T.; Machura, K.; Park, J.K.; Beck, F.X.; Müller, D.N.; Derer, W.; et al. Macrophages regulate salt-dependent volume and blood pressure by a vascular endothelial growth factor-C-dependent buffering mechanism. *Nat. Med.* **2009**, *15*, 545–552. [CrossRef]
45. Machnik, A.; Dahlmann, A.; Kopp, C.; Goss, J.; Wagner, H.; van Rooijen, N.; Eckardt, K.U.; Müller, D.N.; Park, J.K.; Luft, F.C.; et al. Mononuclear phagocyte system depletion blocks interstitial tonicity-responsive enhancer binding protein/vascular endothelial growth factor C expression and induces salt-sensitive hypertension in rats. *Hypertension* **2010**, *55*, 755–761. [CrossRef]
46. Wiig, H.; Schröder, A.; Neuhofer, W.; Jantsch, J.; Kopp, C.; Karlsen, T.V.; Boschmann, M.; Goss, J.; Bry, M.; Rakova, N.; et al. Immune cells control skin lymphatic electrolyte homeostasis and blood pressure. *J. Clin. Investig.* **2013**, *123*, 2803–2815. [CrossRef]
47. Heer, M.; Baisch, F.; Kropp, J.; Gerzer, R.; Drummer, C. High dietary sodium chloride consumption may not induce body fluid retention in humans. *Am. J. Physiol. Renal. Physiol.* **2000**, *278*, F585–F595. [CrossRef]
48. Rakova, N.; Jüttner, K.; Dahlmann, A.; Schröder, A.; Linz, P.; Kopp, C.; Rauh, M.; Goller, U.; Beck, L.; Agureev, A.; et al. Long-term space flight simulation reveals infradian rhythmicity in human Na(+) balance. *Cell Metab.* **2013**, *17*, 125–131. [CrossRef]
49. Kopp, C.; Linz, P.; Wachsmuth, L.; Dahlmann, A.; Horbach, T.; Schöfl, C.; Renz, W.; Santoro, D.; Niendorf, T.; Müller, D.N.; et al. (23)Na magnetic resonance imaging of tissue sodium. *Hypertension* **2012**, *59*, 167–172. [CrossRef]
50. Kopp, C.; Linz, P.; Dahlmann, A.; Hammon, M.; Jantsch, J.; Müller, D.N.; Schmieder, R.E.; Cavallaro, A.; Eckardt, K.U.; Uder, M.; et al. 23Na magnetic resonance imaging-determined tissue sodium in healthy subjects and hypertensive patients. *Hypertension* **2013**, *61*, 635–640. [CrossRef]
51. Schneider, M.P.; Raff, U.; Kopp, C.; Scheppach, J.B.; Toncar, S.; Wanner, C.; Schlieper, G.; Saritas, T.; Floege, J.; Schmid, M.; et al. Skin Sodium Concentration Correlates with Left Ventricular Hypertrophy in CKD. *J. Am. Soc. Nephrol.* **2017**, *28*, 1867–1876. [CrossRef]
52. Dahlmann, A.; Dörfelt, K.; Eicher, F.; Linz, P.; Kopp, C.; Mössinger, I.; Horn, S.; Büschges-Seraphin, B.; Wabel, P.; Hammon, M.; et al. Magnetic resonance-determined sodium removal from tissue stores in hemodialysis patients. *Kidney Int.* **2015**, *87*, 434–441. [CrossRef]
53. Garofalo, C.; Borrelli, S.; Provenzano, M.; De Stefano, T.; Vita, C.; Chiodini, P.; Minutolo, R.; De Nicola, L.; Conte, G. Dietary Salt Restriction in Chronic Kidney Disease: A Meta-Analysis of Randomized Clinical Trials. *Nutrients* **2018**, *10*, 732. [CrossRef] [PubMed]
54. Slagman, M.C.; Waanders, F.; Hemmelder, M.H.; Woittiez, A.J.; Janssen, W.M.; Lambers Heerspink, H.J.; Navis, G.; Laverman, G.D. HOlland NEphrology STudy Group. Moderate dietary sodium restriction added to angiotensin converting enzyme inhibition compared with dual blockade in lowering proteinuria and blood pressure: Randomised controlled trial. *BMJ* **2011**, *343*, d4366. [CrossRef]
55. Vogt, L.; Waanders, F.; Boomsma, F.; de Zeeuw, D.; Navis, G. Effects of dietary sodium and hydrochlorothiazide on the antiproteinuric efficacy of losartan. *J. Am. Soc. Nephrol.* **2008**, *19*, 999–1007. [CrossRef]
56. Kwakernaak, A.J.; Krikken, J.A.; Binnenmars, S.H.; Visser, F.W.; Hemmelder, M.H.; Woittiez, A.J.; Groen, H.; Laverman, G.D.; Navis, G.; Holland Nephrology Study (HONEST) Group. Effects of sodium restriction and hydrochlorothiazide on RAAS blockade efficacy in diabetic nephropathy: A randomised clinical trial. *Lancet Diabetes Endocrinol.* **2014**, *2*, 385–395. [CrossRef]
57. McMahon, E.J.; Bauer, J.D.; Hawley, C.M.; Isbel, N.M.; Stowasser, M.; Johnson, D.W.; Campbell, K.L. A randomized trial of dietary sodium restriction in CKD. *J. Am. Soc. Nephrol.* **2013**, *24*, 2096–2103. [CrossRef] [PubMed]

58. Konishi, Y.; Okada, N.; Okamura, M.; Morikawa, T.; Okumura, M.; Yoshioka, K.; Imanishi, M. Sodium sensitivity of blood pressure appearing before hypertension and related to histological damage in immunoglobulin a nephropathy. *Hypertension* **2001**, *38*, 81–85. [CrossRef]
59. Keyzer, C.A.; van Breda, G.F.; Vervloet, M.G.; de Jong, M.A.; Laverman, G.D.; Hemmelder, M.H.; Janssen, W.M.; Lambers Heerspink, H.J.; Kwakernaak, A.J.; Bakker, S.J.; et al. Effects of Vitamin D Receptor Activation and Dietary Sodium Restriction on Residual Albuminuria in CKD: The ViRTUE-CKD Trial. *J. Am. Soc. Nephrol.* **2017**, *28*, 1296–1305. [CrossRef]
60. Meuleman, Y.; Hoekstra, T.; Dekker, F.W.; Navis, G.; Vogt, L.; van der Boog, P.J.M.; Bos, W.J.W.; van Montfrans, G.A.; van Dijk, S.; ESMO Study Group. Sodium Restriction in Patients With CKD: A Randomized Controlled Trial of Self-management Support. *Am. J. Kidney Dis.* **2017**, *69*, 576–586. [CrossRef]
61. Ruilope, L.M.; Casal, M.C.; Guerrero, L.; Alcázar, J.M.; Férnandez, M.L.; Lahera, V.; Rodicio, J.L. Sodium intake does not influence the effect of verapamil in hypertensive patients with mild renal insufficiency. *Drugs* **1992**, *44* (Suppl. 1), 94–98. [CrossRef]
62. Hwang, J.H.; Chin, H.J.; Kim, S.; Kim, D.K.; Kim, S.; Park, J.H.; Shin, S.J.; Lee, S.H.; Choi, B.S.; Lim, C.S. Effects of intensive low-salt diet education on albuminuria among nondiabetic patients with hypertension treated with olmesartan: A single-blinded randomized, controlled trial. *Clin. J. Am. Soc. Nephrol.* **2014**, *9*, 2059–2069. [CrossRef] [PubMed]
63. de Brito-Ashurst, I.; Perry, L.; Sanders, T.A.; Thomas, J.E.; Dobbie, H.; Varagunam, M.; Yaqoob, M.M. The role of salt intake and salt sensitivity in the management of hypertension in South Asian people with chronic kidney disease: A randomised controlled trial. *Heart* **2013**, *99*, 1256–1260. [CrossRef] [PubMed]
64. Saran, R.; Padilla, R.L.; Gillespie, B.W.; Heung, M.; Hummel, S.L.; Derebail, V.K.; Pitt, B.; Levin, N.W.; Zhu, F.; Abbas, S.R.; et al. A Randomized Crossover Trial of Dietary Sodium Restriction in Stage 3-4 CKD. *Clin. J. Am. Soc. Nephrol.* **2017**, *12*, 399–407. [CrossRef]
65. Minutolo, R.; Borrelli, S.; Chiodini, P.; Scigliano, R.; Bellizzi, V.; Cianciaruso, B.; Nappi, F.; Zamboli, P.; Catapano, F.; Conte, G.; et al. Effects of age on hypertensive status in patients with chronic kidney disease. *J. Hypertens.* **2007**, *25*, 2325–2333. [CrossRef]
66. Kimura, G.; Dohi, Y.; Fukuda, M. Salt sensitivity and circadian rhythm of blood pressure: The keys to connect CKD with cardiovascular events. *Hypertens. Res.* **2010**, *33*, 515–520. [CrossRef]
67. Minutolo, R.; Agarwal, R.; Borrelli, S.; Chiodini, P.; Bellizzi, V.; Nappi, F.; Cianciaruso, B.; Zamboli, P.; Conte, G.; Gabbai, F.B.; et al. Prognostic role of ambulatory blood pressure measurement in patients with nondialysis chronic kidney disease. *Arch. Intern. Med.* **2011**, *171*, 1090–1098. [CrossRef]
68. D'Elia, L.; Rossi, G.; Schiano di Cola, M.; Savino, I.; Galletti, F.; Strazzullo, P. Meta-Analysis of the Effect of Dietary Sodium Restriction with or without Concomitant Renin-Angiotensin-Aldosterone System-Inhibiting Treatment on Albuminuria. *Clin. J. Am. Soc. Nephrol.* **2015**, *10*, 1542–1552. [CrossRef]
69. Borrelli, S.; Leonardis, D.; Minutolo, R.; Chiodini, P.; De Nicola, L.; Esposito, C.; Mallamaci, F.; Zoccali, C.; Conte, G. Epidemiology of CKD Regression in Patients under Nephrology Care. *PLoS ONE* **2015**, *10*, e0140138. [CrossRef]
70. De Nicola, L.; Provenzano, M.; Chiodini, P.; Borrelli, S.; Garofalo, C.; Pacilio, M.; Liberti, M.E.; Sagliocca, A.; Conte, G.; Minutolo, R. Independent Role of Underlying Kidney Disease on Renal Prognosis of Patients with Chronic Kidney Disease under Nephrology Care. *PLoS ONE* **2015**, *10*, e0127071. [CrossRef]
71. Simeoni, M.; Borrelli, S.; Garofalo, C.; Fuiano, G.; Esposito, C.; Comi, A.; Provenzano, M. Atherosclerotic-nephropathy: An updated narrative review. *J. Nephrol.* **2020**. [CrossRef]
72. Abuelo, J.G. Normotensive ischemic acute renal failure. *N. Engl. J. Med.* **2007**, *357*, 797–805. [CrossRef] [PubMed]
73. Minutolo, R.; Borrelli, S.; Scigliano, R.; Bellizzi, V.; Chiodini, P.; Cianciaruso, B.; Nappi, F.; Zamboli, P.; Conte, G.; De Nicola, L. Prevalence and clinical correlates of white coat hypertension in chronic kidney disease. *Nephrol. Dial. Transpl.* **2007**, *22*, 2217–2223. [CrossRef] [PubMed]
74. Minutolo, R.; Gabbai, F.B.; Agarwal, R.; Chiodini, P.; Borrelli, S.; Bellizzi, V.; Nappi, F.; Stanzione, G.; Conte, G.; De Nicola, L. Assessment of achieved clinic and ambulatory blood pressure recordings and outcomes during treatment in hypertensive patients with CKD: A multicenter prospective cohort study. *Am. J. Kidney Dis.* **2014**, *64*, 744–752. [CrossRef] [PubMed]

75. Fagard, R.H.; Staessen, J.A.; Thijs, L.; Gasowski, J.; Bulpitt, C.J.; Clement, D.; de Leeuw, P.W.; Dobovisek, J.; Jääskivi, M.; Leonetti, G.; et al. Response to antihypertensive therapy in older patients with sustained and nonsustained systolic hypertension. Systolic Hypertension in Europe (Syst-Eur) Trial Investigators. *Circulation* **2000**, *102*, 1139–1144. [CrossRef] [PubMed]
76. Merchant, A.; Wald, R.; Goldstein, M.B.; Yuen, D.; Kirpalani, A.; Dacouris, N.; Ray, J.G.; Kiaii, M.; Leipsic, J.; Kotha, V.; et al. Relationship between different blood pressure measurements and left ventricular mass by cardiac magnetic resonance imaging in end-stage renal disease. *J. Am. Soc. Hypertens.* **2015**, *9*, 275–284. [CrossRef]
77. Kalantar-Zadeh, K.; Regidor, D.L.; Kovesdy, C.P.; Van Wyck, D.; Bunnapradist, S.; Horwich, T.B.; Fonarow, G.C. Fluid retention is associated with cardiovascular mortality in patients undergoing long-term hemodialysis. *Circulation* **2009**, *119*, 671–679. [CrossRef]
78. Agarwal, R. Hypervolemia is associated with increased mortality among hemodialysis patients. *Hypertension* **2010**, *56*, 512–517. [CrossRef]
79. Ok, E.; Asci, G.; Chazot, C.; Ozkahya, M.; Mees, E.J. Controversies and problems of volume control and hypertension in haemodialysis. *Lancet* **2016**, *388*, 285–293. [CrossRef]
80. Zoccali, C.; Moissl, U.; Chazot, C.; Mallamaci, F.; Tripepi, G.; Arkossy, O.; Wabel, P.; Stuard, S. Chronic Fluid Overload and Mortality in ESRD. *J. Am. Soc. Nephrol.* **2017**, *28*, 2491–2497. [CrossRef]
81. Cole, N.I.; Swift, P.A.; He, F.J.; MacGregor, G.A.; Suckling, R.J. The effect of dietary salt on blood pressure in individuals receiving chronic dialysis: A systematic review and meta-analysis of randomised controlled trials. *J. Hum. Hypertens.* **2019**, *33*, 319–326. [CrossRef]
82. Mc Causland, F.R.; Waikar, S.S.; Brunelli, S.M. Increased dietary sodium is independently associated with greater mortality among prevalent hemodialysis patients. *Kidney Int.* **2012**, *82*, 204–211. [CrossRef] [PubMed]
83. Van Biesen, W.; Verger, C.; Heaf, J.; IPOD-PD Study Group. Evolution Over Time of Volume Status and PD-Related Practice Patterns in an Incident Peritoneal Dialysis Cohort. *Clin. J. Am. Soc. Nephrol.* **2019**, *14*, 882–893. [CrossRef]
84. Ronco, C.; Verger, C.; Crepaldi, C.; IPOD-PD Study Group. Baseline hydration status in incident peritoneal dialysis patients: The initiative of patient outcomes in dialysis (IPOD-PD study). *Nephrol. Dial. Transpl.* **2015**, *30*, 849–858. [CrossRef] [PubMed]
85. Borrelli, S.; De Nicola, L.; Minutolo, R.; Perna, A.; Provenzano, M.; Argentino, G.; Cabiddu, G.; Russo, R.; La Milia, V.; De Stefano, T.; et al. Sodium toxicity in peritoneal dialysis: Mechanisms and "solutions". *J. Nephrol.* **2020**, *33*, 59–68. [CrossRef] [PubMed]
86. Sun, T.; Sakata, F.; Ishii, T.; Tawada, M.; Suzuki, Y.; Kinashi, H.; Katsuno, T.; Takei, Y.; Maruyama, S.; Mizuno, M.; et al. Excessive salt intake increases peritoneal solute transport rate via local tonicity-responsive enhancer binding protein in subtotal nephrectomized mice. *Nephrol. Dial. Transpl.* **2019**, *34*, 2031–2042. [CrossRef]
87. Dong, J.; Li, Y.; Yang, Z.; Luo, J. Low dietary sodium intake increases the death risk in peritoneal dialysis. *Clin. J. Am. Soc. Nephrol.* **2010**, *5*, 240–247. [CrossRef]
88. Borrelli, S.; La Milia, V.; De Nicola, L.; Cabiddu, G.; Russo, R.; Provenzano, M.; Minutolo, R.; Conte, G.; Garofalo, C.; Study Group Peritoneal Dialysis of Italian Society of Nephrology. Sodium removal by peritoneal dialysis: A systematic review and meta-analysis. *J. Nephrol.* **2019**, *32*, 231–239. [CrossRef]

International Journal of
Molecular Sciences

MDPI

Article

PGI_2 Analog Attenuates Salt-Induced Renal Injury through the Inhibition of Inflammation and Rac1-MR Activation

Daigoro Hirohama [1,2,*], Wakako Kawarazaki [1], Mitsuhiro Nishimoto [1,3], Nobuhiro Ayuzawa [1], Takeshi Marumo [1,4], Shigeru Shibata [1,2] and Toshiro Fujita [1,5]

1 Division of Clinical Epigenetics, Research Center for Advanced Science and Technology, The University of Tokyo, Tokyo 153-8904, Japan; wkawarazaki-tky@umin.ac.jp (W.K.); nishimoto-tky@umin.ac.jp (M.N.); ayuzawa-tky@umin.ac.jp (N.A.); tmarumo-npr@umin.ac.jp (T.M.); shigeru.shibata@med.teikyo-u.ac.jp (S.S.); Toshiro.FUJITA@rcast.u-tokyo.ac.jp (T.F.)

2 Division of Nephrology, Department of Internal Medicine, Teikyo University School of Medicine, Tokyo 173-8606, Japan

3 Department of Internal Medicine, International University of Health and Welfare Mita Hospital, Tokyo 108-8329, Japan

4 Center for Basic Medical Research at Narita Campus, International University of Health and Welfare, Chiba 286-8686, Japan

5 Shinshu University School of Medicine and Research Center for Social Systems, Nagano 389-0111, Japan

* Correspondence: hirohama-tky@umin.ac.jp; Tel.: +81-3-5452-5057

Received: 1 June 2020; Accepted: 18 June 2020; Published: 22 June 2020

Abstract: Renal inflammation is known to be involved in salt-induced renal damage, leading to end-stage renal disease. This study aims to evaluate the role of inflammation in anti-inflammatory and renoprotective effects of beraprost sodium (BPS), a prostaglandin I_2 (PGI_2) analog, in Dahl salt-sensitive (DS) rats. Five-week-old male DS rats were fed a normal-salt diet (0.5% NaCl), a high-salt diet (8% NaCl), or a high-salt diet plus BPS treatment for 3 weeks. BPS treatment could inhibit marked proteinuria and renal injury in salt-loaded DS rats with elevated blood pressure, accompanied by renal inflammation suppression. Notably, high salt increased renal expression of active Rac1, followed by increased Sgk1 expressions, a downstream molecule of mineralocorticoid receptor (MR) signal, indicating salt-induced activation of Rac1-MR pathway. However, BPS administration inhibited salt-induced Rac1-MR activation as well as renal inflammation and damage, suggesting that Rac1-MR pathway is involved in anti-inflammatory and renoprotective effects of PGI_2. Based upon Rac1 activated by inflammation, moreover, BPS inhibited salt-induced activation of Rac1-MR pathway by renal inflammation suppression, resulting in the attenuation of renal damage in salt-loaded DS rats. Thus, BPS is efficacious for the treatment of salt-induced renal injury.

Keywords: blood pressure; inflammation; mineralocorticoid receptor; Rac1; renal injury; salt-sensitive hypertension

1. Introduction

Dietary high-salt intake does not only increase blood pressure but also induce renal injury. Accumulating evidence indicates that inflammation in the kidney plays a key role in salt-induced renal damage, leading to end-stage renal disease [1–3]. N-acetyl-seryl-aspartyl-lysyl-proline, a natural tetrapeptide with anti-inflammatory properties, prevented salt-induced renal damage without affecting the blood pressure in Dahl salt-sensitive (DS) rats [4]. However, it is still unknown how inflammation evoked by a high-salt diet leads to renal injury.

Rac1 is a member of the RhoGTPase subfamily that acts as an intracellular molecular switch, transducing extracellular stimuli to modulate multiple signaling pathways [5]. A signaling cross-talk between mineralocorticoid receptor (MR) and the small GTPase Rac1 as a novel pathway that modulates MR function have been previously identified [6–8]. We have demonstrated that salt loading increases Rac1 activity in the kidneys of DS rats, which is associated with MR activation and upregulation of the MR target gene serum and glucocorticoid-regulated kinase (Sgk1) expression despite reduced circulating levels of aldosterone, a ligand of MR, resulting in salt-induced kidney injury [7]. By contrast, Rac1 and MR activities were appropriately decreased by salt loading in Dahl salt-resistant (DR) and normotensive rats, which were not accompanied by kidney injury [7]. In addition, administration of Rac1 inhibitor NSC23766 suppressed MR activation and the kidney damage induced by salt loading, which was as effective as eplerenone treatment, an MR blocker [7]. Hence, Rac1-MR activation plays a key role in mediating salt-induced kidney injury in DS rats.

Beraprost sodium (BPS) is an orally available and chemically stable prostaglandin I_2 (PGI_2) analog with established safety. It is clinically used to treat pulmonary arterial hypertension [9] and peripheral arterial disease [10]. Several lines of evidence indicate that BPS has the renoprotective effect in various pathological conditions including anti-glomerular basement membrane (GBM) glomerulonephritis [11], obesity-related kidney damage [12], diabetic kidney disease [13,14], unilateral ureteral obstruction [15,16], and contrast-induced nephropathy [17], which is attributed to the anti-inflammatory effect of BPS [11,14,16,18]. BPS also improved survival rates in anti-GBM glomerulonephritis rats and 5/6 nephrectomized chronic kidney disease (CKD) rats [19]. However, the mechanism for the renoprotective effect of BPS is still unknown. Of note, high salt induces renal inflammation in salt-sensitive hypertensive rats [1,2,20], and PGI_2 possesses anti-inflammatory action [11,14,16,18]. Moreover, based upon the previous reports indicating that inflammation activates Rac1 [21–23], there are some possibilities that BPS inhibits salt-induced Rac1-MR activation by inflammation inhibition, resulting in the attenuation of salt-induced renal damage.

These observations led us to the plausible hypothesis that BPS is therapeutically useful for the treatment of salt-induced renal damage through the suppression of activated Rac1-MR pathway. To test the hypothesis in this study, we investigated the renoprotective effect of BPS in the DS rat, which is a commonly used model of salt-sensitive hypertension [24].

2. Results

2.1. BPS Treatment Did Not Alter Blood Pressure Levels in High-Salt-Fed DS Rats

All animals completed the study protocol. Male DS rats received a normal-salt (0.5% NaCl, NS) diet, high-salt (8% NaCl, HS) diet, or high-salt diet plus BPS treatment (HS-BPS) for 3 weeks. All rats were randomly assigned to NS, HS, or HS-BPS group.

There were no significant changes in body weight after high-salt feeding with or without BPS treatment (Figure 1A). High-salt feeding increased urine sodium excretion at 3 weeks; however, BPS did not have any effect on sodium excretion (Figure 1B). Systolic blood pressure levels were similar among NS, HS, and HS-BPS rats at baseline (Figure 1C,D). BPS treatment slightly, but insignificantly, decreased blood pressure levels (Figure 1C,E). Heart weight to body weight ratios, the marker of cardiac hypertrophy, were higher in HS rats compared with NS rats (Figure 1F). These ratios remained unchanged by BPS treatment (Figure 1F).

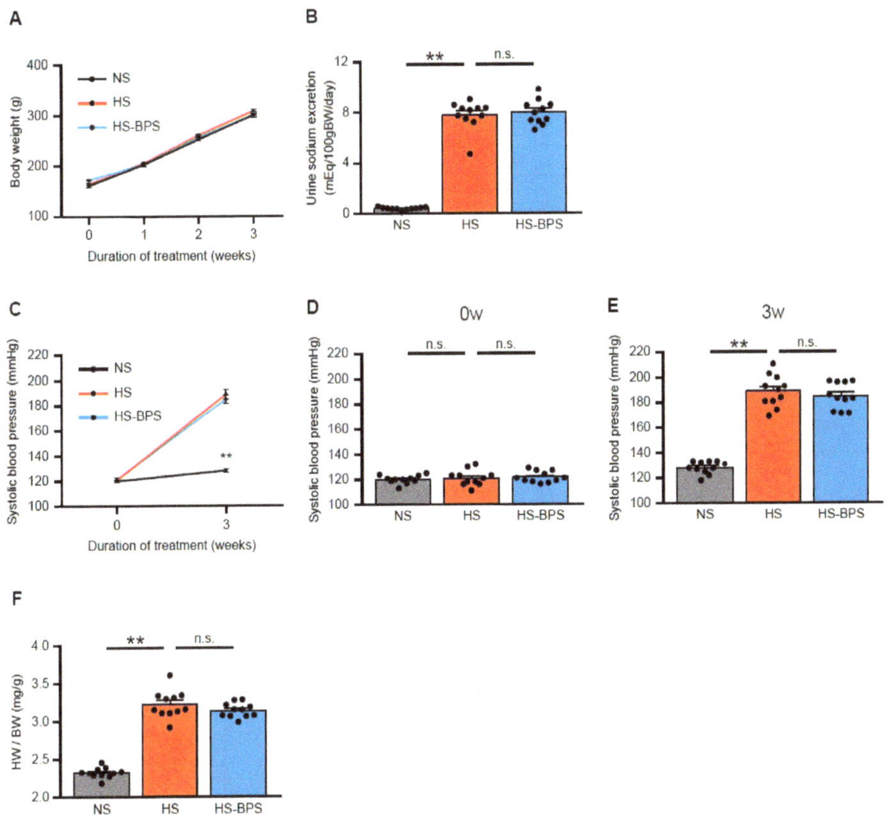

Figure 1. Effects of BPS on blood pressure levels in high-salt-fed DS rats. (**A**) Change in body weight, (**B**) urine sodium excretion levels at 3 weeks, (**C–E**) systolic blood pressure levels at 0 and 3 weeks, and (**F**) heart weight to body weight ratio of DS rats on a normal-salt (0.5% NaCl, NS) diet, high-salt (8% NaCl, HS) diet or high-salt diet plus BPS treatment (HS-BPS) for 3 weeks (n = 11 per group). The asterisks in (**C**) correspond to NS vs. HS group at 3 weeks. Data are expressed as mean ± SEM. ** $p < 0.01$; n.s., not significant.

2.2. Administration of BPS Ameliorates Proteinuria and Renal Injury in High-Salt-Fed DS Rats

We measured the urine protein excretion levels at 3 weeks to evaluate whether BPS exerted protective effects on renal injury in HS rats. HS rats showed the overt increase in urine protein excretion (Figure 2A,B). Of interest, urine protein excretion was markedly reduced by BPS treatment (Figure 2A,B).

To determine whether BPS ameliorated renal injury, we also addressed renal histology in periodic acid–Schiff (PAS)-stained kidney sections. HS rats displayed glomerulosclerosis and tubulointerstitial injury manifested by vacuolation and desquamation of the renal epithelial cells, accompanied by proteinaceous cast formation (Figure 2C,D), in agreement with previous reports [7,25]. Our preliminary results showed that there was very little fibrosis in HS rats, indicating that HS rats have salt-induced kidney injury in early stage. Semiquantitative evaluation of renal histology demonstrated that BPS significantly attenuated glomerular and tubulointerstitial damages (Figure 2C,D). Renal histology also revealed the strong correlation between glomerular and tubulointerstitial damages in HS and HS-BPS rats (r = 0.80, $p < 0.01$) (Supplementary Figure S1A), indicating that BPS treatment attenuated tubulointerstitial damages along with the mitigation of glomerular damages. Moreover,

BPS significantly reduced serum creatinine levels in high-salt-fed DS rats (Supplementary Figure S1B). BPS also decreased blood urea nitrogen (BUN) levels, however, the decrease was not statistically significant (HS: 24.4 ± 0.9 vs. HS-BPS: 22.4 ± 0.5 mg/dL; $p = 0.065$) (Supplementary Figure S1C).

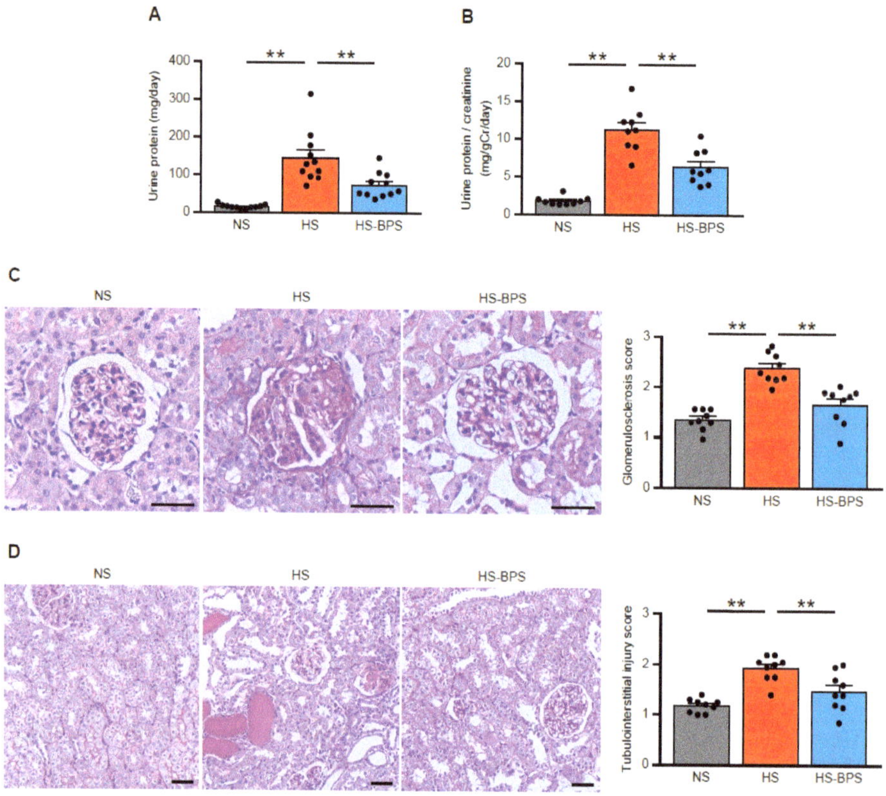

Figure 2. BPS administration ameliorates proteinuria and renal injury in high-salt-fed DS rats. (**A**) Levels of urine protein excretion at 3 weeks and (**B**) urine protein per creatinine excretion in NS, HS, and HS-BPS rats (n = 11 per group). (**C**) Representative photomicrographs of period acid–Schiff (PAS)-stained kidney sections and quantification of glomerulosclerosis (see also Methods; n = 9 per group). Scale bars, 50 μm. (**D**) Representative photomicrographs of PAS-stained kidney sections and quantification of tubulointerstitial injury (see also Methods; n = 9 per group). Scale bars, 50 μm. Data are expressed as mean ± SEM. ** $p < 0.01$.

2.3. BPS Reduced Renal MR Pathway Activation via Rac1 Activity Suppression in High-Salt-Fed DS Rats

We next explored the possible mechanism of the renoprotective effects observed in HS-BPS rats. Accumulating evidence suggests that MR and its ligand, aldosterone, play a pivotal role in the progression of kidney injury [26–28], including salt-induced kidney injury [7,25,29].

Thus, we evaluated renin-angiotensin-aldosterone system (RAAS) in our animal models. High-salt feeding suppressed plasma renin activity, angiotensin II concentrations, and serum aldosterone concentrations (Figure 3A–C), indicating that RAAS was suppressed by high-salt feeding. In spite of suppressed aldosterone levels, HS rats demonstrated increased expressions of Sgk1 (Figure 3D), a downstream molecule of MR signaling, indicating MR activation in HS rats.

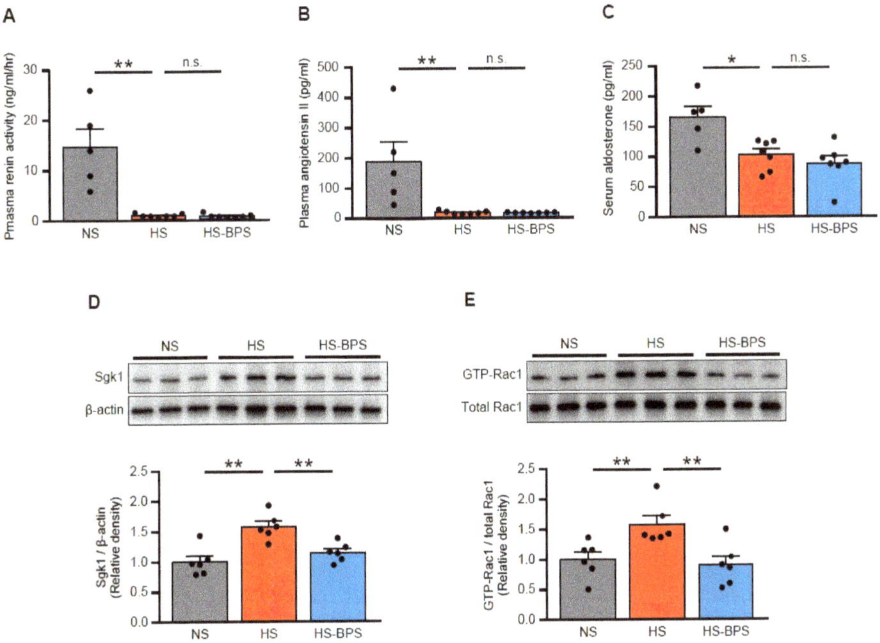

Figure 3. BPS reduced renal MR pathway activation through Rac1 activity suppression in high-salt-fed DS rats. (**A**) Plasma renin activity, (**B**) plasma angiotensin II concentration, and (**C**) serum aldosterone concentration in NS, HS, and HS-BPS rats ($n = 5$ for NS, $n = 7$ for HS, $n = 7$ for HS-BPS rats). (**D**) Western blot analysis of MR downstream effector Sgk1 in the renal cortex. Blots show biological replicates, and bar graphs show the results of quantitation ($n = 6$ per group). (**E**) Western blot analysis of GTP-bound Rac1 in the renal cortex. Blots show biological replicates, and bar graphs show quantitation results ($n = 6$ per group). Data are expressed as mean ± SEM. * $p < 0.05$; ** $p < 0.01$; n.s., not significant.

With regard to the mechanism of salt-induced MR activation, we previously identified the role of Rac1 as a modulator of MR activity [6–8]. We investigated Rac1 activity in the renal cortex of HS rats to confirm whether renal Rac1 is activated. HS rats showed increased expressions of GTP-Rac1 (Figure 3E), an active form of Rac1, consistent with previous findings [7].

BPS treatment suppressed MR signaling as assessed by reduced Sgk1 expressions (Figure 3D), despite unchanged serum aldosterone levels (Figure 3C), indicating that MR signaling was ligand independently regulated. In addition, renal Rac1 activity was suppressed by BPS administration. These results suggested that BPS reduced MR overactivation through renal Rac1 activity suppression.

2.4. BPS Alleviates Renal Inflammation in High-Salt-Fed DS Rats

We next investigated the factors inducing renal Rac1 activation in our model. Previous studies documented the role of inflammation that is responsible for Rac1 activation [21–23]. Therefore, we quantitatively analyzed the gene expression of several cytokines. Quantitative real-time RT-PCR revealed that the expression of pro-inflammatory cytokines including interleukin-1β (*IL-1β*), tumor necrosis factor-α (*TNF-α*), interleukin-6 (*IL-6*), plasminogen activator inhibitor-1 (*PAI-1/SERPINE1*), and monocyte chemoattractant protein-1 (*MCP-1/CCL2*) were significantly increased by high-salt feeding (Figure 4A–E). Moreover, HS rats also showed increased expression of *CD68* (Figure 4F), a marker of macrophage expression. We measured IL-1β in proteins of renal cortex by enzyme-linked immunosorbent assay (ELISA) to validate the gene expression. We found elevated IL-1β levels in renal proteins of HS rats (Figure 4G). BPS administration significantly reduced all of these pro-inflammatory cytokine gene expressions and IL-1β protein expressions (Figure 4A–G), indicating that inflammation in the kidney of high-salt-fed DS rats was alleviated by BPS treatment.

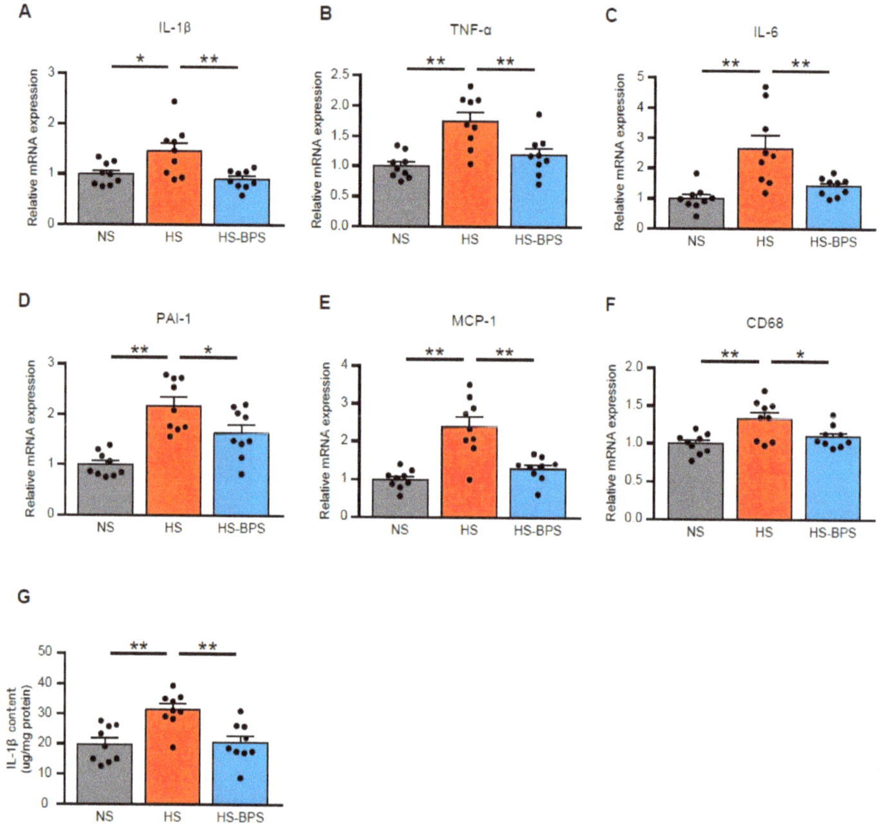

Figure 4. BPS alleviates renal inflammation in high-salt-fed DS rats. Quantitative analysis of (**A**) *IL-1β*, (**B**) *TNF-α*, (**C**) *IL-6*, (**D**) *PAI-1/SERPINE1*, (**E**) *MCP-1/CCL2*, and (**F**) *CD68* gene expression in the renal cortex by real-time RT-PCR ($n = 9$ per group). (**G**) IL-1β content in renal cortex evaluated by ELISA ($n = 9$ per group). Data are expressed as mean ± SEM. * $p < 0.05$; ** $p < 0.01$.

3. Discussion

Using DS rats as a model of salt-sensitive hypertension, this study demonstrated that BPS counteracts against the progression of salt-induced kidney injury. High-salt diet induced overt proteinuria, accompanied by glomerulosclerosis and tubulointerstitial injury in DS rats. High-salt-fed DS rats showed increased expressions of active Rac1 and Sgk1, a downstream molecule of MR signaling, indicating Rac1-MR pathway activation, associated with elevated renal inflammation. BPS administration attenuated proteinuria and renal injury. Moreover, Rac1-MR activation and inflammation in the kidney of high-salt-fed DS rats were ameliorated by BPS treatment, which suggested that inflammation-induced Rac1-MR pathway activation is involved in the progression of salt-induced kidney injury and that BPS treatment suppresses renal inflammation, leading to the attenuation of Rac1-MR activation and kidney damage (Figure 5).

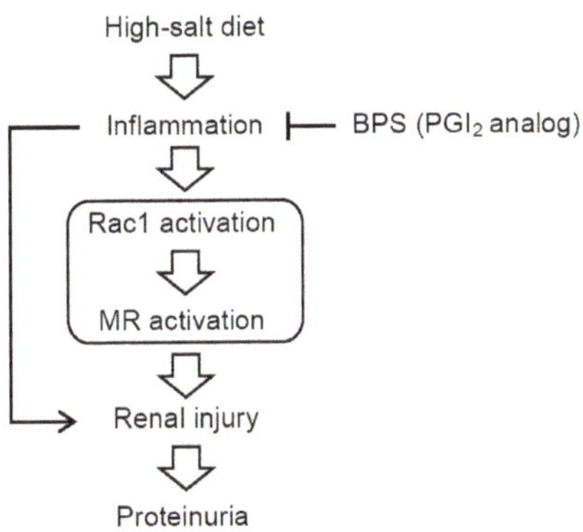

Figure 5. Schematic diagram illustrating the hypothesis that Rac1-MR pathway activation by inflammation is involved in the progression of renal injury in high-salt-fed DS rats. In high-salt-fed DS rats, inflammation-induced Rac1-MR pathway activation is involved in the progression of renal injury and massive proteinuria. Treatment of BPS, a PGI_2 analog, suppresses inflammation, leading to the reduction of Rac1-MR activation and kidney damage.

In this study, we used DS rats that serve as an excellent model of salt-sensitive hypertension and associated kidney injury, exhibiting many phenotypic characteristics common in human hypertension [24]. Increasing evidence suggests the role of inflammation in the progression of chronic kidney disease [30,31]. Furthermore, salt-sensitive hypertension in human and experimental animal models has been demonstrated to be accompanied by progressive kidney damage leading to end-stage renal disease, which is associated with elevated inflammation [1–3].

We speculate that there are several possibilities explaining the mechanisms whereby BPS treatment had renoprotective effects in this model. First, BPS can exert anti-inflammatory effects in salt-induced kidney injury. Accumulating evidence shows that BPS has renoprotective effects in various experimental kidney disease models [11–17,19]. Indeed, the observed renal protective effects of BPS in this study were associated with the reduction of inflammation. These data are in line with previous reports showing anti-inflammatory roles of BPS [11,14,16,18].

A second possibility is that BPS treatment reduced renal injury through the suppression of Rac1-MR pathway activation in the kidney. We have demonstrated that salt loading increases Rac1 activity in the kidneys of DS rats, which is associated with MR activation, resulting in salt-induced kidney injury [7]. However, in this previous study, it remained undetermined what induced Rac1 activation. Many investigators have evaluated factors modulating Rac1 activity. Some studies reported that Rac1 can be activated by inflammatory cytokines [21–23], dietary salt [6,7], angiotensin II [32,33], angiotensin II with salt [34], aldosterone [26], high glucose [35], reactive oxygen species [36], and mechanical stress [37]. Of note, the anti-inflammatory effect of BPS was prominent in this study. Therefore, it is possible that BPS suppressed renal Rac1-MR activation through the reduction of inflammation in the kidney.

Third, BPS might decrease blood pressure. BPS has been used for the treatment of pulmonary arterial hypertension [9] and peripheral arterial disease [10]. Although BPS has a vasodilatory effect, it is not an antihypertensive drug. Indeed, hypertension is a major risk factor for chronic kidney disease progression, which can also occur as a consequence of a progressive decline in renal function [38]. In the present study, three weeks of BPS treatment slightly, but insignificantly, decreased blood pressure by tail-cuff method. In the further study, it is important to evaluate continuous blood pressure measured by radiotelemetry.

The Rho GTPases (Rac1, RhoA, and Cdc42) act as molecular switches that regulate actin dynamics [39], and consequently play a pivotal role in maintaining the cytoskeletal and molecular integrity of the podocyte foot processes in a dynamic manner [40]. Changes of activity of these GTPases lead to hypo- or hyper-motility of podocytes, resulting in proteinuria [40,41]. Therefore, Rho GTPases have drawn attention as potential therapeutic applications in CKD. We previously demonstrated that high-salt feeding induced hypertension and podocyte injury in DS rats [25]. In this study, eplerenone, a MR antagonist, and hydralazine reduced blood pressure to the similar extent in high-salt-fed DS rats; however, podocyte injury and urine protein excretion were ameliorated only in eplerenone-treated group [25]. These findings raised the possibility that the reduction of urine protein by BPS treatment in the current study was mediated via the suppression of Rac1-MR pathway activation in podocytes.

With respect to the clinical application of BPS for the treatment of moderate to severe CKD patients, phase II clinical trial showed that TRK-100 STP (sustained-release BPS) significantly prevented the estimated glomerular filtration rate reduction in patients with non-diabetic CKD patients [42], but Phase III (CASSIOPEIR) trial did not prove a beneficial effect in CKD progression [43]. Another phase III trial of aldosterone antagonist, spironolactone, in patients with preserved cardiac function heart failure (TOPCAT) did not achieve a significant reduction in the primary composite outcome of death from cardiovascular causes, aborted cardiac arrest, or hospitalization for the management of heart failure [44]. However, in a sub-analysis of this trial, an unusually large difference was identified in the placebo event rates between the sites conducting TOPCAT in the four countries in America compared with those in Russia and Georgia [45]. To explain the regional difference, investigators measured metabolite concentrations of spironolactone and found significant regional discrepancies in the reported use and the actual use of spironolactone [46]. These results imply that medication adherence is important to achieve therapeutic goals, and that a sub-analysis of CASSIOPEIR trial according to BPS itself or metabolite of BPS concentrations is needed. Moreover, a sub-analysis study to estimate dietary salt intake in individual patients is also needed, since high salt activate Rac1-MR pathway in hypertensive CKD patients [47].

Prostaglandins appear when arachidonic acid is released from the plasma membrane by phospholipases and metabolized by the peroxidase actions of cyclooxygenases to prostaglandin H_2, which can be thereafter converted into more stable biologically active prostaglandins, including PGI_2 and prostaglandin E_2 (PGE_2) [48,49]. Prostaglandins exert various functions in the pathology and physiology of kidney, in which the levels of prostaglandins can be regulated at multiple steps [48,49]. Several investigators reported that inhibition of prostaglandin production with either nonselective or selective inhibitors of cyclooxygenase-2 (COX-2) activity can induce or exacerbate salt-sensitive hypertension [50–52]. Notably, the protective effect of PGI_2 activity against the development of atherothrombotic cardiovascular disease has been demonstrated to be mediated by the inhibition of various cellular processes, including platelet activation, leukocyte adhesion, as well as vascular smooth muscle cell modulation [53]. Consistently, salt-loaded DS rats showed lower urine excretion of 6-keto PGF1α, a metabolite of PGI_2, as compared to salt-loaded DR rats [54], suggesting that decreased production of PGI_2 in the kidney contribute to the development of salt-sensitive hypertension, although we did not measure these metabolites in this study. With respect to the relationship between prostaglandins and salt-sensitive hypertension, moreover, a recent study reveals that COX-2 derived PGE_2 in macrophages plays an important role in both kidney and skin in maintaining homeostasis in response to chronically increased dietary salt [55]. Therefore, this study also implies that inhibiting COX-2 expression or activity in macrophages can result in a predisposition to salt-sensitive hypertension [55]. Thus, it is possible that prostaglandins in macrophages play roles in the development of salt-sensitive hypertension and subsequent salt-induced renal injury in our model, which is a subject for future study.

A limitation of our study is that the exact mechanisms whereby BPS suppresses Rac1-MR activation remain undetermined. Direct demonstration by cell culture experiments are needed to clarify the mechanisms, which was not addressed in this study. It is also unknown whether BPS elicits primary protective effects in the kidney. Given that the renoprotective effect of BPS was evaluated only in male rats, the result may not apply to female rats. Despite these limitations, this study clearly demonstrates that BPS has renoprotective effects in salt-induced kidney injury. Given our data, we speculate that anti-inflammatory effects of BPS reduced Rac1-MR activation in the kidney, leading to the attenuation of renal damage. Our data indicate that BPS can be a therapeutic option to treat CKD, especially in patients with early stage of CKD. Additional prospective clinical studies are needed to further address this hypothesis.

4. Materials and Methods

4.1. Animals and Experimental Design

Animal care and treatment complied with the standards described in the Guidelines for the Care and Use of Laboratory Animals of the University of Tokyo (Tokyo, Japan). All studies were approved by the Institutional Animal Care and Use Committee of the University of Tokyo (RAC 140202, date: 1 July 2014). Five-week-old male DS rats were purchased from Japan SLC (Shizuoka, Japan), which were randomly divided into three groups as follows: a normal-salt (0.5% NaCl) diet group (NS, n = 11), a high-salt (8% NaCl) diet group (HS, n = 11), and a high-salt diet plus BPS (provided by Toray Industries, Inc., Tokyo, Japan, 750 mg/kg/day in drinking water), a PGI_2 analog, treatment group (HS-BPS, n = 11). The dosages of BPS used were determined according to the renoprotective effects in previous studies [12,19]. The rats were fed either a normal-salt (MF diet, Oriental Yeast, Tokyo, Japan) or a high-salt (MF diet containing 8% NaCl, Oriental Yeast) diet for 3 weeks. The NS group was used as control. Body weight was recorded every week during the experimental period. All rats had free access to drinking water and food under temperature-controlled conditions and a 12-h light/dark cycle.

4.2. Blood Pressure Measurements in Conscious Rats

The systolic blood pressures of conscious rats were measured at 3 weeks using the tail-cuff method (BP-98A; Softron, Tokyo, Japan), as previously described [7,56]. Measurements were performed at daytime and the average of five serial measurements taken in a calm state was calculated for each rat. A dark cover was placed over animals to reduce stress.

4.3. Metabolic Studies

Twenty-four-hour urine samples were collected using an individual metabolic cage (Natsume, Tokyo, Japan) at 3 weeks. Urine protein and creatinine levels were measured at SRL (Tokyo, Japan).

4.4. Blood Collection and Laboratory Measurements

At the end of the experiments, we extracted blood from the inferior vena cava with syringes under pentobarbital anesthesia. Blood was immediately transferred into a blood collection tube containing EDTA-2Na and centrifuged at 5000 rpm for 20 min at 4 °C; then plasma was removed. The remaining blood volume was transferred into a blood collection tube containing serum-separating medium and centrifuged at 5000 rpm for 20 min at 4 °C; then serum was removed. Plasma and serum were stored at −30 °C until analyses. Plasma renin activity, plasma angiotensin II concentrations, and serum aldosterone concentrations were determined by radioimmunoassay (SRL). Serum creatinine and blood urea nitrogen levels were measured at SRL.

4.5. Renal Histology

Kidneys were harvested and fixed in 4% paraformaldehyde overnight at 4 °C and embedded in paraffin. Subsequently, 3-μm-thick tissue sections were stained with PAS reagent. Pathological changes in kidney tissues were observed under a light microscope (Leica DMI 4000B, Leica Microsystems, Wetzlar, Germany). We semiquantitatively assessed the degrees of glomerular damage and tubulointerstitial injury according to an established scoring system [6,7,26]. For evaluation of glomerulosclerosis, glomeruli were scored on a scale of 0 to 4, according to the following criteria: 0 normal; 1, involvement of 1–25% of the glomerular tufts; 2 involvement of 26–50% of the glomerular tufts; 3, involvement of 51–75% of the glomerular tufts; and 4, involvement of 75–100% of the glomerular tufts. Fifteen glomeruli

(×200) of each kidney were scored and the mean value was calculated as the glomerulosclerosis score. Tubulointerstitial injury was defined as tubular cast formation, tubular dilatation, tubular atrophy, or inflammatory cell infiltration. The extent of damage was scored 0 to 4, according to the following criteria: 0, normal; 1, involvement of 1–25% of the cortex; 2, involvement of 26–50% of the cortex; 3, involvement of 51–75% of the cortex; and 4, involvement of 75–100% of the cortex. Ten cortical fields (×100) of each kidney were scored and the mean value was defined as the tubulointerstitial injury score. A blind evaluation of the glomerulosclerosis and tubulointerstitial injury was done by two renal pathologists.

4.6. Western Blot Analysis

Kidneys were removed, snap frozen in liquid nitrogen, and stored at −80 °C until homogenization. Kidneys were homogenized on ice with extraction buffer containing 50 mM Tris-HCl (pH 8.0), 150 mM NaCl, 1% NP-40, 0.5% sodium deoxycholate, 0.1% SDS, and protease inhibitors (Complete, Roche Diagnostics, Basel, Switzerland) and were centrifuged at 14000 rpm at 4 °C for 30 min to obtain the cellular proteins in the supernatant. Protein concentrations were determined using a BCA protein assay (Fujifilm Wako Pure Chemical Corporation, Osaka, Japan).

Western blotting (WB) was performed as previously described [57], with some modifications. Briefly, equal amounts of protein were mixed with 2× Laemmli sample buffer, boiled for 10 min, separated on polyacrylamide gels, and transferred to polyvinylidene fluoride (PVDF) membranes. The membranes were blocked with PVDF-blocking reagent (Toyobo, Osaka, Japan) for 30 min at room temperature and incubated with primary and peroxidase-conjugated secondary antibodies. Signals were detected using the ECL Prime Western Blotting Detection Reagent (GE Healthcare, Waukesha, WI, USA) and scanned using ImageQuant LAS 4000 mini (GE Healthcare). Signal intensity was quantitated using ImageJ 1.46r software (National Institutes of Health, Bethesda, MD, USA).

4.7. Quantitative RT-PCR Analysis

Total RNA was isolated from kidneys using an RNeasy mini kit (Qiagen, Venlo, Netherlands) according to the manufacturer's instructions. RNA quantity and purity were assessed via Nanodrop 2000 spectrophotometer (Thermo Scientific, Waltham, MA, USA). Total RNA having OD 260/280 ratio between 2.0 and 2.2 was used for reverse transcription. cDNA was synthesized using RevatraAce reverse transcriptase (Toyobo) according to the manufacturer's instructions. Quantitative RT-PCR analyses were performed using a StepOnePlus Real-Time PCR System (Applied Biosystems, Waltham, MA, USA), as described previously [58]. The expression levels of *TNF-α*, *PAI-1/SERPINE1*, *MCP-1/CCL2*, and glyceraldehyde 3-phosphate dehydrogenase (*GAPDH*) were then analyzed using the TaqMan Universal PCR Master Mix (Applied Biosystems). TaqMan primer/probes sets (Applied Biosystems) were used, and the GenBank accession number and assay ID are as follow: *TNF-α* (NM_012675.3, RN01525859_g1), *PAI-1/SERPINE1* (NM_012620.1, RN01481341_m1), *MCP-1/CCL2* (NM_031530.1, RN00580555_m1), and *GAPDH* (NM_017008.4, Rn01775763_g1). SYBR Green PCR Master Mix (Applied Biosystems) was used with primers for detection of other genes (Supplementary Table S1). Denaturation took place at 95 °C for 15 s and annealing and extension at 60 °C for 1 min for 40 cycles. The comparative cycle threshold method was used to compare gene expression levels. Expression levels were normalized against the housekeeping gene *GAPDH*.

4.8. IL-1β ELISA

Renal IL-1β protein concentrations were determined by enzyme-linked immunosorbent assay (rat IL-1β/IL-1F2 Quantikine ELISA, RLB00, R&D Systems, Minneapolis, MN, USA). Kidney was completely homogenized in an extraction buffer containing 10 mM Tris-HCl (pH 7.8), 150 mM NaCl, 1% NP40, 1 mM EDTA, and protease inhibitors (Complete, Roche Diagnostics). After homogenization, samples were centrifuged at 4 °C, 14,000 rpm for 30 min. The clean supernatant was then used to determine IL-1β protein concentration, according to the manufacturer's protocol.

4.9. Antibodies

Primary antibodies used in WB studies included those for Sgk1 (SAB2104902, 1:6000; Sigma-Aldrich, St. Louis, MO, USA), β-actin (ab8227, 1:5000; Abcam, Cambridge, UK), GTP-Rac1 (#26903, 1:3000; NewEast Biosciences, Malvern, PA, USA), and total Rac1 (#05-389, 1:6000; Millipore, Billerica, MA, USA).

4.10. Statistical Analyses

Data are expressed as mean ± SE. For comparison across multiple groups, one-way or two-way ANOVA followed by a Tukey–Kramer post hoc test was performed. $p < 0.05$ was considered statistically significant. Statistical analyses were performed with GraphPad Prism 7 (GraphPad Software, La Jolla, CA, USA).

Supplementary Materials: The following are available online at http://www.mdpi.com/1422-0067/21/12/4433/s1.

Author Contributions: Conceptualization, D.H. and T.F.; methodology, D.H. and T.F.; software, D.H.; validation and formal analysis, D.H. and T.F.; investigation, D.H.; data curation, D.H.; writing and original draft preparation, D.H.; writing and review and editing, W.K., M.N., N.A., T.M., S.S., and T.F.; visualization, D.H.; supervision, T.F.; project administration, D.H. and T.F.; funding acquisition, D.H. and T.F. All authors have read and agreed to the final version of the manuscript.

Funding: This work was supported in part by Japan Society for the Promotion of Science (JSPS) KAKENHI grants 19K17732 (to D.H.) and 15H05788 (to T.F.). The study was also supported by the Japan Foundation for Applied Enzymology (to D.H.).

Acknowledgments: We thank Toray Industries, Inc. for providing BPS. We also thank Atsushi Watanabe for performing pathological analyses.

Conflicts of Interest: The authors declare no conflict of interest.

Abbreviations

BPS	beraprost sodium
CKD	chronic kidney disease
DR rats	Dahl salt-resistant rats
DS rats	Dahl salt-sensitive rats
ELISA	enzyme-linked immunosorbent assay
GBM	glomerular basement membrane
IL-1β	interleukin-1β
IL-6	interleukin-6
MCP-1	monocyte chemoattractant protein-1
MR	mineralocorticoid receptor
PAI-1	plasminogen activator inhibitor-1
PAS	periodic acid–Schiff
RAAS	renin-angiotensin-aldosterone system
Sgk1	serum and glucocorticoid-regulated kinase
TNF-α	tumor necrosis factor-α

References

1. Tian, N.; Gu, J.W.; Jordan, S.; Rose, R.A.; Hughson, M.D.; Manning, R.D., Jr. Immune suppression prevents renal damage and dysfunction and reduces arterial pressure in salt-sensitive hypertension. *Am. J. Physiol. Heart Circ. Physiol.* **2007**, *292*, H1018–H1025. [CrossRef] [PubMed]
2. Lu, X.; Crowley, S.D. Inflammation in Salt-Sensitive Hypertension and Renal Damage. *Curr. Hypertens. Rep.* **2018**, *20*, 103. [CrossRef] [PubMed]
3. Hirohama, D.; Fujita, T. Evaluation of the pathophysiological mechanisms of salt-sensitive hypertension. *Hypertens. Res.* **2019**, *42*, 1848–1857. [CrossRef] [PubMed]

4. Worou, M.E.; Liao, T.D.; D'Ambrosio, M.; Nakagawa, P.; Janic, B.; Peterson, E.L.; Rhaleb, N.E.; Carretero, O.A. Renal protective effect of N-acetyl-seryl-aspartyl-lysyl-proline in dahl salt-sensitive rats. *Hypertension* **2015**, *66*, 816–822. [CrossRef] [PubMed]
5. Nagase, M.; Fujita, T. Role of Rac1-mineralocorticoid-receptor signalling in renal and cardiac disease. *Nat. Rev. Nephrol.* **2013**, *9*, 86–98. [CrossRef] [PubMed]
6. Shibata, S.; Nagase, M.; Yoshida, S.; Kawarazaki, W.; Kurihara, H.; Tanaka, H.; Miyoshi, J.; Takai, Y.; Fujita, T. Modification of mineralocorticoid receptor function by Rac1 GTPase: Implication in proteinuric kidney disease. *Nat. Med.* **2008**, *14*, 1370–1376. [CrossRef]
7. Shibata, S.; Mu, S.; Kawarazaki, H.; Muraoka, K.; Ishizawa, K.; Yoshida, S.; Kawarazaki, W.; Takeuchi, M.; Ayuzawa, N.; Miyoshi, J.; et al. Rac1 GTPase in rodent kidneys is essential for salt-sensitive hypertension via a mineralocorticoid receptor-dependent pathway. *J. Clin. Investig.* **2011**, *121*, 3233–3243. [CrossRef]
8. Fujita, T. Mechanism of salt-sensitive hypertension: Focus on adrenal and sympathetic nervous systems. *J. Am. Soc. Nephrol.* **2014**, *25*, 1148–1155. [CrossRef]
9. Nagaya, N.; Uematsu, M.; Okano, Y.; Satoh, T.; Kyotani, S.; Sakamaki, F.; Nakanishi, N.; Miyatake, K.; Kunieda, T. Effect of orally active prostacyclin analogue on survival of outpatients with primary pulmonary hypertension. *J. Am. Coll. Cardiol.* **1999**, *34*, 1188–1192. [CrossRef]
10. Lievre, M.; Morand, S.; Besse, B.; Fiessinger, J.N.; Boissel, J.P. Oral Beraprost sodium, a prostaglandin I(2) analogue, for intermittent claudication: A double-blind, randomized, multicenter controlled trial. Beraprost et Claudication Intermittente (BERCI) Research Group. *Circulation* **2000**, *102*, 426–431. [CrossRef]
11. Yamada, M.; Sasaki, R.; Sato, N.; Suzuki, M.; Tamura, M.; Matsushita, T.; Kurumatani, H. Amelioration by beraprost sodium, a prostacyclin analogue, of established renal dysfunction in rat glomerulonephritis model. *Eur. J. Pharmacol.* **2002**, *449*, 167–176. [CrossRef]
12. Sato, N.; Kaneko, M.; Tamura, M.; Kurumatani, H. The prostacyclin analog beraprost sodium ameliorates characteristics of metabolic syndrome in obese Zucker (fatty) rats. *Diabetes* **2010**, *59*, 1092–1100. [CrossRef] [PubMed]
13. Watanabe, M.; Nakashima, H.; Mochizuki, S.; Abe, Y.; Ishimura, A.; Ito, K.; Fukushima, T.; Miyake, K.; Ogahara, S.; Saito, T. Amelioration of diabetic nephropathy in OLETF rats by prostaglandin I(2) analog, beraprost sodium. *Am. J. Nephrol.* **2009**, *30*, 1–11. [CrossRef] [PubMed]
14. Peng, L.; Li, J.; Xu, Y.; Wang, Y.; Du, H.; Shao, J.; Liu, Z. The Protective Effect of Beraprost Sodium on Diabetic Nephropathy by Inhibiting Inflammation and p38 MAPK Signaling Pathway in High-Fat Diet/Streptozotocin-Induced Diabetic Rats. *Int. J. Endocrinol.* **2016**, *2016*, 1690474. [CrossRef] [PubMed]
15. Takenaka, M.; Machida, N.; Ida, N.; Satoh, N.; Kurumatani, H.; Yamane, Y. Effect of beraprost sodium (BPS) in a new rat partial unilateral ureteral obstruction model. *Prostaglandins Leukot. Essent. Fatty Acids* **2009**, *80*, 263–267. [CrossRef] [PubMed]
16. Li, S.; Wang, Y.; Chen, L.; Wang, Z.; Liu, G.; Zuo, B.; Liu, C.; Sun, D. Beraprost sodium mitigates renal interstitial fibrosis through repairing renal microvessels. *J. Mol. Med.* **2019**, *97*, 777–791. [CrossRef] [PubMed]
17. Yano, T.; Itoh, Y.; Kubota, T.; Sendo, T.; Koyama, T.; Fujita, T.; Saeki, K.; Yuo, A.; Oishi, R. A prostacyclin analog prevents radiocontrast nephropathy via phosphorylation of cyclic AMP response element binding protein. *Am. J. Pathol.* **2005**, *166*, 1333–1342. [CrossRef]
18. Fujiwara, K.; Nagasaka, A.; Nagata, M.; Yamamoto, K.; Imamura, S.; Oda, N.; Sawai, Y.; Hayakawa, N.; Suzuki, A.; Itoh, M. A stable prostacyclin analogue reduces high serum TNF-alpha levels in diabetic patients. *Exp. Clin. Endocrinol. Diabetes* **2004**, *112*, 390–394. [CrossRef]
19. Yamaguchi, S.; Inada, C.; Tamura, M.; Sato, N.; Yamada, M.; Itaba, S.; Okazaki, S.; Matsuura, H.; Fujii, S.; Matsuda, F.; et al. Beraprost sodium improves survival rates in anti-glomerular basement membrane glomerulonephritis and 5/6 nephrectomized chronic kidney disease rats. *Eur. J. Pharmacol.* **2013**, *714*, 325–331. [CrossRef]
20. Zhu, Q.; Li, X.X.; Wang, W.; Hu, J.; Li, P.L.; Conley, S.; Li, N. Mesenchymal stem cell transplantation inhibited high salt-induced activation of the NLRP3 inflammasome in the renal medulla in Dahl S rats. *Am. J. Physiol. Ren. Physiol.* **2016**, *310*, F621–F627. [CrossRef]
21. Uddin, S.; Lekmine, F.; Sharma, N.; Majchrzak, B.; Mayer, I.; Young, P.R.; Bokoch, G.M.; Fish, E.N.; Platanias, L.C. The Rac1/p38 mitogen-activated protein kinase pathway is required for interferon alpha-dependent transcriptional activation but not serine phosphorylation of Stat proteins. *J. Biol. Chem.* **2000**, *275*, 27634–27640. [PubMed]

22. Woo, C.H.; Eom, Y.W.; Yoo, M.H.; You, H.J.; Han, H.J.; Song, W.K.; Yoo, Y.J.; Chun, J.S.; Kim, J.H. Tumor necrosis factor-alpha generates reactive oxygen species via a cytosolic phospholipase A2-linked cascade. *J. Biol. Chem.* **2000**, *275*, 32357–32362. [CrossRef] [PubMed]
23. Schuringa, J.J.; Dekker, L.V.; Vellenga, E.; Kruijer, W. Sequential activation of Rac-1, SEK-1/MKK-4, and protein kinase Cdelta is required for interleukin-6-induced STAT3 Ser-727 phosphorylation and transactivation. *J. Biol. Chem.* **2001**, *276*, 27709–27715. [CrossRef]
24. Wadei, H.M.; Textor, S.C. The role of the kidney in regulating arterial blood pressure. *Nat. Rev. Nephrol.* **2012**, *8*, 602–609. [CrossRef] [PubMed]
25. Nagase, M.; Shibata, S.; Yoshida, S.; Nagase, T.; Gotoda, T.; Fujita, T. Podocyte injury underlies the glomerulopathy of Dahl salt-hypertensive rats and is reversed by aldosterone blocker. *Hypertension* **2006**, *47*, 1084–1093. [CrossRef]
26. Shibata, S.; Nagase, M.; Yoshida, S.; Kawachi, H.; Fujita, T. Podocyte as the target for aldosterone: Roles of oxidative stress and Sgk1. *Hypertension* **2007**, *49*, 355–364. [CrossRef] [PubMed]
27. Briet, M.; Schiffrin, E.L. Aldosterone: Effects on the kidney and cardiovascular system. *Nat. Rev. Nephrol.* **2010**, *6*, 261–273. [CrossRef]
28. Shibata, S.; Ishizawa, K.; Uchida, S. Mineralocorticoid receptor as a therapeutic target in chronic kidney disease and hypertension. *Hypertens. Res.* **2017**, *40*, 221–225. [CrossRef]
29. Kawarazaki, H.; Ando, K.; Nagae, A.; Fujita, M.; Matsui, H.; Fujita, T. Mineralocorticoid receptor activation contributes to salt-induced hypertension and renal injury in prepubertal Dahl salt-sensitive rats. *Nephrol. Dial. Transplant.* **2010**, *25*, 2879–2889. [CrossRef]
30. Ruiz-Ortega, M.; Rayego-Mateos, S.; Lamas, S.; Ortiz, A.; Rodrigues-Diez, R.R. Targeting the progression of chronic kidney disease. *Nat. Rev. Nephrol.* **2020**, *16*, 269–288. [CrossRef]
31. Furman, D.; Campisi, J.; Verdin, E.; Carrera-Bastos, P.; Targ, S.; Franceschi, C.; Ferrucci, L.; Gilroy, D.W.; Fasano, A.; Miller, G.W.; et al. Chronic inflammation in the etiology of disease across the life span. *Nat. Med.* **2019**, *25*, 1822–1832. [CrossRef] [PubMed]
32. Takemoto, M.; Node, K.; Nakagami, H.; Liao, Y.; Grimm, M.; Takemoto, Y.; Kitakaze, M.; Liao, J.K. Statins as antioxidant therapy for preventing cardiac myocyte hypertrophy. *J. Clin. Investig.* **2001**, *108*, 1429–1437. [CrossRef] [PubMed]
33. Nishida, M.; Tanabe, S.; Maruyama, Y.; Mangmool, S.; Urayama, K.; Nagamatsu, Y.; Takagahara, S.; Turner, J.H.; Kozasa, T.; Kobayashi, H.; et al. G alpha 12/13- and reactive oxygen species-dependent activation of c-Jun NH2-terminal kinase and p38 mitogen-activated protein kinase by angiotensin receptor stimulation in rat neonatal cardiomyocytes. *J. Biol. Chem.* **2005**, *280*, 18434–18441. [CrossRef] [PubMed]
34. Kawarazaki, W.; Nagase, M.; Yoshida, S.; Takeuchi, M.; Ishizawa, K.; Ayuzawa, N.; Ueda, K.; Fujita, T. Angiotensin II- and salt-induced kidney injury through Rac1-mediated mineralocorticoid receptor activation. *J. Am. Soc. Nephrol.* **2012**, *23*, 997–1007. [CrossRef]
35. Yoshida, S.; Ishizawa, K.; Ayuzawa, N.; Ueda, K.; Takeuchi, M.; Kawarazaki, W.; Fujita, T.; Nagase, M. Local mineralocorticoid receptor activation and the role of Rac1 in obesity-related diabetic kidney disease. *Nephron Exp. Nephrol.* **2014**, *126*, 16–24. [CrossRef]
36. Nagase, M.; Ayuzawa, N.; Kawarazaki, W.; Ishizawa, K.; Ueda, K.; Yoshida, S.; Fujita, T. Oxidative stress causes mineralocorticoid receptor activation in rat cardiomyocytes: Role of small GTPase Rac1. *Hypertension* **2012**, *59*, 500–506. [CrossRef]
37. Ayuzawa, N.; Nagase, M.; Ueda, K.; Nishimoto, M.; Kawarazaki, W.; Marumo, T.; Aiba, A.; Sakurai, T.; Shindo, T.; Fujita, T. Rac1-Mediated Activation of Mineralocorticoid Receptor in Pressure Overload-Induced Cardiac Injury. *Hypertension* **2016**, *67*, 99–106. [CrossRef]
38. Townsend, R.R.; Taler, S.J. Management of hypertension in chronic kidney disease. *Nat. Rev. Nephrol.* **2015**, *11*, 555–563. [CrossRef]
39. Haga, R.B.; Ridley, A.J. Rho GTPases: Regulation and roles in cancer cell biology. *Small GTPases* **2016**, *7*, 207–221. [CrossRef]
40. Perico, L.; Conti, S.; Benigni, A.; Remuzzi, G. Podocyte-actin dynamics in health and disease. *Nat. Rev. Nephrol.* **2016**, *12*, 692–710. [CrossRef]
41. Ashraf, S.; Kudo, H.; Rao, J.; Kikuchi, A.; Widmeier, E.; Lawson, J.A.; Tan, W.; Hermle, T.; Warejko, J.K.; Shril, S.; et al. Mutations in six nephrosis genes delineate a pathogenic pathway amenable to treatment. *Nat. Commun.* **2018**, *9*, 1960. [CrossRef]

42. Koyama, A.; Fujita, T.; Gejyo, F.; Origasa, H.; Isono, M.; Kurumatani, H.; Okada, K.; Kanoh, H.; Kiriyama, T.; Yamada, S. Orally active prostacyclin analogue beraprost sodium in patients with chronic kidney disease: A randomized, double-blind, placebo-controlled, phase II dose finding trial. *BMC Nephrol.* **2015**, *16*, 165. [CrossRef]
43. Nakamoto, H.; Yu, X.Q.; Kim, S.; Origasa, H.; Zheng, H.; Chen, J.; Joo, K.W.; Sritippayawan, S.; Chen, Q.; Chen, H.C.; et al. Effects of Sustained-Release Beraprost in Patients With Primary Glomerular Disease or Nephrosclerosis: CASSIOPEIR Study Results. *Ther. Apher. Dial.* **2020**, *24*, 42–55. [CrossRef]
44. Pitt, B.; Pfeffer, M.A.; Assmann, S.F.; Boineau, R.; Anand, I.S.; Claggett, B.; Clausell, N.; Desai, A.S.; Diaz, R.; Fleg, J.L.; et al. Spironolactone for heart failure with preserved ejection fraction. *N. Engl. J. Med.* **2014**, *370*, 1383–1392. [CrossRef] [PubMed]
45. Pfeffer, M.A.; Claggett, B.; Assmann, S.F.; Boineau, R.; Anand, I.S.; Clausell, N.; Desai, A.S.; Diaz, R.; Fleg, J.L.; Gordeev, I.; et al. Regional variation in patients and outcomes in the Treatment of Preserved Cardiac Function Heart Failure With an Aldosterone Antagonist (TOPCAT) trial. *Circulation* **2015**, *131*, 34–42. [CrossRef] [PubMed]
46. de Denus, S.; O'Meara, E.; Desai, A.S.; Claggett, B.; Lewis, E.F.; Leclair, G.; Jutras, M.; Lavoie, J.; Solomon, S.D.; Pitt, B.; et al. Spironolactone Metabolites in TOPCAT-New Insights into Regional Variation. *N. Engl. J. Med.* **2017**, *376*, 1690–1692. [CrossRef]
47. Nishimoto, M.; Ohtsu, H.; Marumo, T.; Kawarazaki, W.; Ayuzawa, N.; Ueda, K.; Hirohama, D.; Kawakami-Mori, F.; Shibata, S.; Nagasc, M.; et al. Mineralocorticoid receptor blockade suppresses dietary salt-induced ACEI/ARB-resistant albuminuria in non-diabetic hypertension: A sub-analysis of evaluate study. *Hypertens. Res.* **2019**, *42*, 514–521. [CrossRef]
48. Hao, C.M.; Breyer, M.D. Physiological regulation of prostaglandins in the kidney. *Annu. Rev. Physiol.* **2008**, *70*, 357–377. [CrossRef]
49. Ricciotti, E.; FitzGerald, G.A. Prostaglandins and inflammation. *Arterioscler. Thromb. Vasc. Biol.* **2011**, *31*, 986–1000. [CrossRef] [PubMed]
50. Hernanz, R.; Briones, A.M.; Salaices, M.; Alonso, M.J. New roles for old pathways? A circuitous relationship between reactive oxygen species and cyclo-oxygenase in hypertension. *Clin. Sci.* **2014**, *126*, 111–121. [CrossRef]
51. Cheng, H.F.; Harris, R.C. Renal effects of non-steroidal anti-inflammatory drugs and selective cyclooxygenase-2 inhibitors. *Curr. Pharm. Des.* **2005**, *11*, 1795–1804. [CrossRef] [PubMed]
52. Yu, Y.; Ricciotti, E.; Scalia, R.; Tang, S.Y.; Grant, G.; Yu, Z.; Landesberg, G.; Crichton, I.; Wu, W.; Pure, E.; et al. Vascular COX-2 modulates blood pressure and thrombosis in mice. *Sci. Transl. Med.* **2012**, *4*, 132ra154. [CrossRef] [PubMed]
53. Stitham, J.; Midgett, C.; Martin, K.A.; Hwa, J. Prostacyclin: An inflammatory paradox. *Front. Pharmacol.* **2011**, *2*, 24. [CrossRef]
54. Falardeau, P.; Martineau, A. In vivo production of prostaglandin I2 in Dahl salt-sensitive and salt-resistant rats. *Hypertension* **1983**, *5*, 701–705. [CrossRef]
55. Zhang, M.Z.; Yao, B.; Wang, Y.; Yang, S.; Wang, S.; Fan, X.; Harris, R.C. Inhibition of cyclooxygenase-2 in hematopoietic cells results in salt-sensitive hypertension. *J. Clin. Investig.* **2015**, *125*, 4281–4294. [CrossRef]
56. Mu, S.; Shimosawa, T.; Ogura, S.; Wang, H.; Uetake, Y.; Kawakami-Mori, F.; Marumo, T.; Yatomi, Y.; Geller, D.S.; Tanaka, H.; et al. Epigenetic modulation of the renal beta-adrenergic-WNK4 pathway in salt-sensitive hypertension. *Nat. Med.* **2011**, *17*, 573–580. [CrossRef] [PubMed]
57. Hirohama, D.; Ayuzawa, N.; Ueda, K.; Nishimoto, M.; Kawarazaki, W.; Watanabe, A.; Shimosawa, T.; Marumo, T.; Shibata, S.; Fujita, T. Aldosterone Is Essential for Angiotensin II-Induced Upregulation of Pendrin. *J. Am. Soc. Nephrol.* **2018**, *29*, 57–68. [CrossRef] [PubMed]
58. Marumo, T.; Yagi, S.; Kawarazaki, W.; Nishimoto, M.; Ayuzawa, N.; Watanabe, A.; Ueda, K.; Hirahashi, J.; Hishikawa, K.; Sakurai, H.; et al. Diabetes Induces Aberrant DNA Methylation in the Proximal Tubules of the Kidney. *J. Am. Soc. Nephrol.* **2015**, *26*, 2388–2397. [CrossRef]

International Journal of
Molecular Sciences

MDPI

Article

Na^+-Coupled Nutrient Cotransport Induced Luminal Negative Potential and Claudin-15 Play an Important Role in Paracellular Na^+ Recycling in Mouse Small Intestine

Michiko Nakayama [1,†], Noriko Ishizuka [1,†], Wendy Hempstock [1], Akira Ikari [2] and Hisayoshi Hayashi [1,*]

1 Laboratory of Physiology, School of Food and Nutritional Sciences, University of Shizuoka, Yada 52-1, Suruga-ku, Shizuoka 422-8526, Japan; m-7ka8ma@outlook.jp (M.N.); n-ishizuka@u-shizuoka-ken.ac.jp (N.I.); w.hempstock@gmail.com (W.H.)
2 Laboratory of Biochemistry, Department of Biopharmaceutical Sciences, Gifu Pharmaceutical University, Gifu 501-1196, Japan; ikari@gifu-pu.ac.jp
* Correspondence: hayashih@u-shizuoka-ken.ac.jp; Tel.: +81-54-264-5532
† These authors contributed equally to this work.

Received: 6 December 2019; Accepted: 30 December 2019; Published: 7 January 2020

Abstract: Many nutrients are absorbed via Na^+ cotransport systems, and therefore it is predicted that nutrient absorption mechanisms require a large amount of luminal Na^+. It is thought that Na^+ diffuses back into the lumen via paracellular pathways to support Na^+ cotransport absorption. However, direct experimental evidence in support of this mechanism has not been shown. To elucidate this, we took advantage of claudin-15 deficient (*cldn15*$^{-/-}$) mice, which have been shown to have decreased paracellular Na^+ permeability. We measured glucose-induced currents (ΔI_{sc}) under open- and short-circuit conditions and simultaneously measured changes in unidirectional $^{22}Na^+$ fluxes (ΔJ^{Na}) in Ussing chambers. Under short-circuit conditions, application of glucose resulted in an increase in ΔI_{sc} and unidirectional mucosal to serosal $^{22}Na^+$ ($\Delta J^{Na}{}_{MS}$) flux in both wild-type and *cldn15*$^{-/-}$ mice. However, under open-circuit conditions, ΔI_{sc} was observed but $\Delta J^{Na}{}_{MS}$ was strongly inhibited in wild-type but not in *cldn15*$^{-/-}$ mice. In addition, in the duodenum of mice treated with cholera toxin, paracellular Na^+ conductance was decreased and glucose-induced $\Delta J^{Na}{}_{MS}$ increment was observed under open-circuit conditions. We concluded that the Na^+ which is absorbed by Na^+-dependent glucose cotransport is recycled back into the lumen via paracellular Na^+ conductance through claudin-15, which is driven by Na^+ cotransport induced luminal negativity.

Keywords: tight junction; Na^+ cotransport; leaky epithelia

1. Introduction

Nutrient absorption in the small intestine is essential for assimilation of nutrients required for energy and growth. To meet these requirements, nutrients are efficiently absorbed from the luminal side, which is the external milieu. In nutrient absorbing cells, many nutrients cross the luminal membrane via specific transporters which require cotransport with luminal Na^+. Na^+ coupling allows nutrients to be transported against their concentration gradient from a low luminal concentration to a higher intracellular concentration. The driving force for nutrient transporters is provided by the electrochemical Na^+ gradient across the luminal membrane. This Na^+ gradient is produced by the Na-K-ATPase on the basolateral membrane which keeps the intracellular Na^+ concentration low. Therefore, it is expected that Na^+ nutrient cotransport concomitantly occurs with net Na^+ absorption from the luminal (extracellular) to the serosal side [1].

There are many Na^+ nutrient cotransport systems in the small intestine, such as glucose, amino acids, etc. [2–4]. It is, therefore, envisaged that Na^+-dependent nutrient absorption mechanisms require a large amount of luminal Na^+, which should be theoretically predictable as follows: For a healthy adult male, daily energy intake is 2500 kcal. The percentage of energy derived from the three major macronutrients in a typical Western diet is carbohydrates (52%), fat (33%), and protein (15%) [5]. Since protein and carbohydrates yield 4 kcal/g and 9 kcal/g for fat, the total amount of daily intake of carbohydrates, fat, and protein is about 325, 92, and 93 g, respectively. The resultant products of digestion produce large amounts of monosaccharides and amino acids in the lumen. The intake of 325 g of carbohydrates will yield approximately 1.8 moles of monosaccharide, which is mostly composed of glucose. The primary transporter that mediates glucose transport in the intestinal brush border membrane has been identified as Na^+-dependent glucose transporter SGLT1, which operates with a transport stoichiometry of 2 Na^+:1 glucose [6,7]. Thus, it is estimated that 3.6 moles of Na^+ are needed for the absorption of glucose only, which corresponds to 23 L of isotonic NaCl solution, containing 210 g NaCl. This volume of fluid is approximately two times larger than that of extracellular fluid, which is 20% of body weight. With regards to protein, assuming that the average molecular weight of an amino acid residue in protein is 110, i.e., 93 g of protein will yield approximately 0.8 moles of amino acids, which needs an equivalent amount of luminal Na^+ for amino acid absorption from the luminal side. Taking into consideration all of the Na^+-dependent nutrient absorption, nutrient absorption mechanisms would require a large amount of luminal Na^+.

How does the small intestine meet the requirements for such a large amount of Na^+ for absorption of nutrients? One possible source is digestive juices. In humans, it is thought that 9L/day of isotonic fluid enters the lumen of the proximal small intestine through diet and secretion of the upper digestive tract [8]. This fluid is composed of 2 L from diet, 1 L of saliva, 2 L of gastric juice, 1 L of bile, 2 L of pancreatic juice, and 1 L of secretions from the small intestine, which contain only 0.8 moles of Na^+ in total. Another luminal Na^+ providing mechanism would be via the paracellular pathway. It is well known that small intestinal epithelia are classified as leaky epithelia, which means its paracellular conductance is ~90% or more of the total tissue conductance and it is cation selective ($P_{Na} > P_{Cl}$) [9]. However, the physiological relevance of cationic selectivity of the paracellular pathway remains to be fully elucidated. The properties of the paracellular pathway are dependent on tight junctions, which occur where epithelial cells are closely connected to each other. The claudin family of tight junction proteins is critical in determining the paracellular ionic permeability and selectivity. The claudin family consists of 27 integral membrane proteins [10]. The subcellular distribution of the claudins varies; while claudin-2 and -15 are exclusively in the tight junctions, other isoforms, e.g., claudin-4 and -7, are found in the basolateral membrane [11–13]. This diverging pattern of distribution suggests that individual claudins are engaged in different physiological functions. We previously showed that a loss of claudin-15 decreased the luminal Na^+ concentration and glucose absorption is inhibited in mouse small intestine [14]. It is hypothesized that Na^+ diffuses back into the lumen via the paracellular pathway to support nutrient absorption [15]. However, direct experimental evidence in support of this idea has not been shown. In this study, to investigate whether paracellular Na^+ conductance through claudin-15 is involved in this Na^+ recycling system and to elucidate the role of Na^+-nutrient cotransport induced luminal negativity for Na^+ recycling, we measured glucose-induced short-circuit currents (ΔI_{sc}) under open- and short-circuit conditions in Ussing chambers. In addition, we simultaneously measured changes in unidirectional mucosal to serosal $^{22}Na^+$ ($\Delta J^{Na}{}_{MS}$) flux in wild-type mice and compared them with those of 15 deficient (*cldn15*$^{-/-}$) mice. Furthermore, to understand the mechanism of oral rehydration therapy, which is based on the notion that the Na^+ that is absorbed by Na^+-glucose cotransport enters into systemic circulation [16], we measured glucose-induced unidirectional $\Delta J^{Na}{}_{MS}$ in cholera toxin-diarrhea model mice. The results showed that under the short-circuit conditions in wild-type mice, luminal application of glucose resulted in an increase in $\Delta J^{Na}{}_{MS}$ which corresponded to the amplitude of ΔI_{sc}. However, under open-circuit conditions, a ΔI_{sc} increase was observed but $\Delta J^{Na}{}_{MS}$ was strongly inhibited. These results suggest that Na^+ is recycled back to the lumen under physiological conditions. In *cldn15*$^{-/-}$ mice, a robust increase in $\Delta J^{Na}{}_{MS}$ was observed under open-circuit conditions, suggesting that the efficiency of Na^+-recycling systems was reduced. This phenomenon was also mimicked by cholera toxin-induced diarrhea in wild-type mice.

Our study demonstrates that the Na^+ which is absorbed by Na^+-nutrient cotransport is recycled back into the lumen via paracellular Na^+ conductance through claudin-15, which is driven by Na^+ cotransport induced luminal potential.

2. Results

2.1. Baseline Na^+ Absorption Mechanisms in Wild-Type Mice

Baseline I_{sc} and $^{22}Na^+$ unidirectional fluxes were measured simultaneously in the same preparations in wild-type mice (Table 1).

Table 1. Basal $^{22}Na^+$ flux and electrical parameters in wild-type mice.

	J^{Na}, μmol/cm²/h			I_{sc}, μmol/cm²/h	G_t, mS/cm²	n
	M→S	S→M	Net			
	Short-Circuit Conditions					
Control	51.4 ± 2.3	24.6 ± 1.7	26.9 ± 1.5	2.4 ± 0.5	58.7±2.2	4
S3226	38.9 ± 3.4 *	28.3 ± 1.9	10.6 ± 3.9 *	1.7 ± 0.2	54.6±2.8	6
	Open-Circuit Conditions					
Control	44.2 ± 2.6 N.S.	22.8 ± 1.6 N.S.	21.4 ± 3.7 N.S.	1.8 ± 0.3 N.S.	55.2±2.4 N.S.	3

10 μM S3336 was added to the mucosal side. Each value represents the mean ± SE. * $p < 0.05$ as compared with control. N.S. not significant as compared with short-circuit conditions by Mann–Whitney test. M→S indicates the unidirectional mucosal to serosal Na^+ flux. S→M indicates the unidirectional serosal to mucosal Na^+ flux. n: Number of animals examined.

The unidirectional mucosal to serosal $^{22}Na^+$ flux ($J^{Na}{}_{MS}$: 51.4 ± 2.3 μmol/cm²/h) was larger than the serosal to mucosal flux ($J^{Na}{}_{SM}$: 24.6 ± 1.7 μmol/cm²/h). This result suggests that Na^+ absorption occurred in the baseline conditions. The magnitude of the net $^{22}Na^+$ flux ($J^{Na}{}_{Net}$: 26.9 ± 1.5 μmol/cm²/h) was significantly greater than that of the basal short-circuit current (I_{sc}) (2.4 ± 0.5 μmol/cm²/h) suggesting that the net Na^+ absorption occurs mostly via an electroneutral Na^+/H^+ exchange mechanism. To determine the contribution of Na^+/H^+ exchanger-3 isoform (NHE3) to baseline I_{sc} and $^{22}Na^+$ unidirectional fluxes, we used the NHE3 specific inhibitor S3226. In the presence of the S3226, the basal net Na^+ flux was decreased by 60% ($J^{Na}{}_{Net}$: 10.6 ± 3.9 μmol/cm²/h). Basal I_{sc} and transmural tissue conductance (G_t) were not significantly changed by S3226 ($p = 0.29$ and 0.25, I_{sc} and G_t, respectively), suggesting that paracellular ion permeability is not affected by S3226. However, 10 μM S3226 did not completely inhibit basal Na^+ absorption. Although other NHE isoforms could be involved in basal Na^+ absorption, these results suggest that the basal net Na^+ absorption is mainly dependent on NHE3 transport, consistent with what has been previously reported [17].

2.2. Activation of SGLT1 Concomitantly Increases Mucosal to Serosal $^{22}Na^+$ Fluxes under Short-Circuit Conditions

As shown in Figure 1A, the addition of glucose to the mucosal side increased I_{sc} (ΔI_{sc} 13.7 ± 0.8 μmol/cm²/h) in wild-type mice. $J^{Na}{}_{MS}$ was also significantly increased (Figure 1B, $\Delta J^{Na}{}_{MS}$, 12.5 ± 0.8 μmol/cm²/h, $n = 5$) after luminal application of glucose, while the unidirectional serosal to mucosal $^{22}Na^+$ flux ($J^{Na}{}_{SM}$) was not significantly changed after the addition of luminal glucose (Figure 1B, 25.5 ± 1.1 vs. 23.5 ± 1.1 μmol/cm²/h, $p = 0.21$, before and after the addition of glucose, respectively).

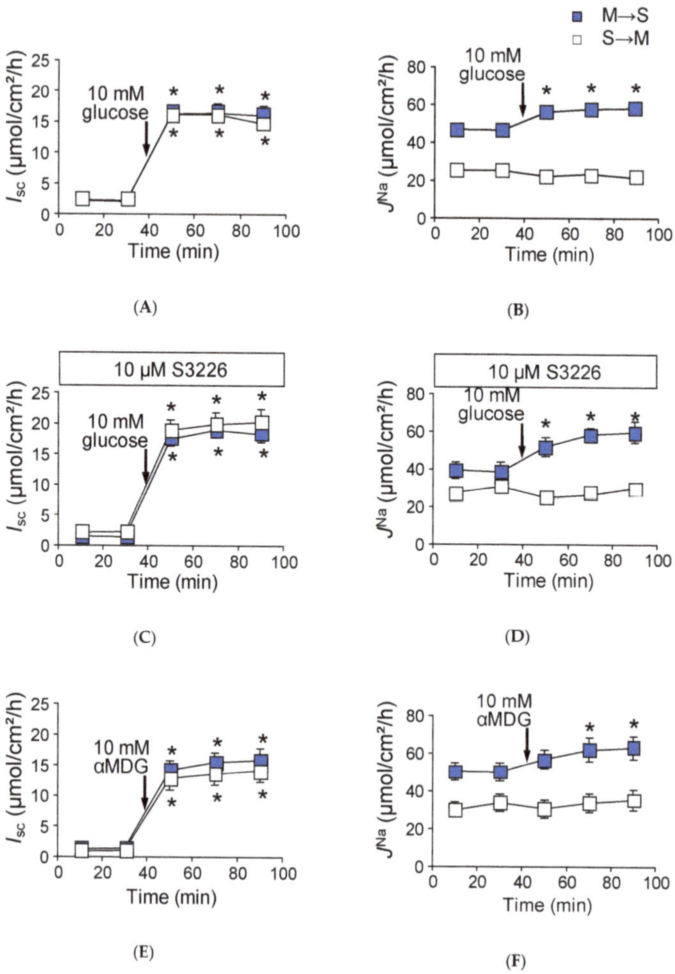

Figure 1. Activation of SGLT1 increases unidirectional mucosal to serosal $^{22}Na^+$ fluxes under short-circuit conditions in wild-type mice: Glucose-induced short-circuit current changes (I_{sc}) (**A**) and $^{22}Na^+$ unidirectional flux changes (J^{Na}) (**B**) were measured simultaneously in Ussing chambers, as described in the Materials and Methods. After measure basal I_{sc} and J^{Na} during the initial 30 min (squares represent mean of 9 and 8 measurements mucosal to serosal (M to S) and serosal to mucosal (S to M), respectively), glucose was added to the mucosal side, indicated by arrows ($n = 9$ and 8, M to S and S to M, respectively). The effects of S3226 on glucose-induced I_{sc} (**C**), and J^{Na} (**D**). Thirty minutes before initiation of measurement, 10 μM S3226 was added to the mucosal side ($n = 5$ and 5, M to S and S to M, respectively). Non-metabolizable sugar alpha methyl-D-glucose (αMDG) increase of I_{sc} (**E**) and J^{Na} (**F**) ($n = 6$ and 6, M to S and S to M, respectively). Closed squares indicate mucosal to serosal unidirectional $^{22}Na^+$ fluxes ($J^{Na}{}_{MS}$) and open squares indicate mucosal to serosal $^{22}Na^+$ fluxes ($J^{Na}{}_{SM}$). Each point represents the mean ± SE. Where error bars are absent, they are smaller than the symbol used. * $p < 0.05$ as compared with the baseline control.

These results suggest that glucose-induced $\Delta J^{Na}{}_{MS}$ is mediated by the Na^+-dependent glucose transporter SGLT1. To confirm this, we conducted four experiments. First, the specific SGLT1 inhibitor phloridzin (0.2 mM) was added to the luminal side, and glucose-induced $\Delta J^{Na}{}_{MS}$ was measured. In the presence of phloridzin, both glucose-induced ΔI_{sc} and ΔJ^{Na}_{MS} increments were totally abolished (I_{sc}: 1.1 ± 0.3 vs. −0.1 ± 0.3 μmol/cm²/h, p = 0.06, J^{Na}_{MS}: 48.8 ± 4.2 vs. 46.1 ± 1.9 μmol/cm²/h, p = 0.88, n = 3 before and after addition of glucose, respectively). Second, transepithelial $^{36}Cl^-$ unidirectional flux was measured with or without luminal glucose. It is thought that Na^+-coupled glucose transport from the lumen to intercellular spaces provides an osmotic gradient that results in passive ion movement through tight junctions [18]. However, there was no discernable changes in $^{36}Cl^-$ unidirectional fluxes with or without luminal glucose (ΔJ^{Cl}_{Net}: 14.5 ± 1.8 vs. 14.0 ± 1.7 μmol/cm²/h, p = 0.54, n = 5 before and after addition of glucose, respectively). We next assessed the contribution of NHE3 to glucose-induced ΔJ^{Na}_{MS} increments, as Na^+-coupled glucose uptake stimulates NHE3 transport activity in the mouse jejunum [19]. The above-mentioned glucose-induced ΔJ^{Na}_{MS} increments could be mediated by NHE3 and not SGLT1. To examine this possibility, we measured the glucose-induced $^{22}Na^+$ unidirectional fluxes in the presence of the NHE3 specific inhibitor S3226 [20]. As shown in Figure 1C, the addition of glucose to the mucosal side resulted in an increase of the I_{sc} (ΔI_{sc}: 17.5 ± 1.6 μmol/cm²/h, n = 5), which is slightly higher in the absence of S3226 (p = 0.05). Robust glucose-induced ΔJ^{Na}_{MS} increment was also observed in the presence of S3226 (Figure 1D, ΔJ^{Na}_{MS}: 20.2 ± 1.8 μmol/cm²/h), suggesting that NHE3 is not responsible for glucose-induced $^{22}Na^+$ unidirectional flux increments. Finally, we assessed whether glucose metabolic pathways contribute to ΔJ^{Na}_{MS} increments or not. The non-metabolizable glucose analogue α-methyl-D-glucose (αMDG) was used instead of D-glucose, and the αMDG-induced $^{22}Na^+$ unidirectional fluxes were measured. The addition of αMDG to the mucosal side increased the I_{sc} in a dose-dependent manner. This change in I_{sc} conformed to Michaelis–Menten kinetics, and these values were not significantly different as compared with those of glucose (V_{max}: 551 ± 47 vs. 661 ± 45 μA/cm², p = 0.14, K_m: 10.9 ± 2.9 vs. 5.1 ± 1.2 mM, p = 0.14, glucose and αMDG, respectively). As shown in Figure 1E,F, the addition of 10 mM αMDG to the mucosal side increased the I_{sc} (ΔI_{sc}: 12.7 ± 1.7 μmol/cm²/h) and ΔJ^{Na}_{MS} (12.3 ± 1.6 μmol/cm²/h). These values are not significantly different as compared with those of glucose values (p = 0.55, 0.89, ΔI_{sc} and ΔJ^{Na}_{MS}, respectively). Taken together, these results suggest that glucose-induced increment of ΔJ^{Na}_{MS} is mediated by SGLT1.

We next assessed the quantitative relationship between ΔI_{sc} and ΔJ^{Na}_{Net} under short-circuit conditions, where ΔJ^{Na}_{Net} is plotted as a function of ΔI_{sc} (Figure 2, closed circles).

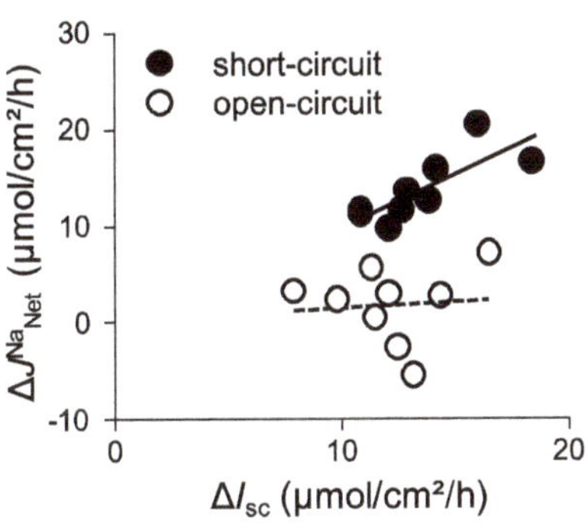

Figure 2. The relationship between changes of glucose-induced I_{sc} (ΔI_{sc}) and changes of glucose-induced net $^{22}Na^+$ fluxes (ΔJ^{Na}_{Net}) in wild-type mice: Glucose-induced ΔI_{sc} and net Na^+ flux (J^{Na}_{Net}) were calculated from the data of Figure 1 (short-circuit conditions) and Figure 3 (open-circuit conditions) and replotted. ΔI_{sc} was determined by subtracting baseline values from those obtained after addition of glucose. Mean values for the last two periods after addition of glucose are taken as the change in I_{sc} and J^{Na}. Net Na^+ flux (J^{Na}_{Net}) was calculated using adjacent tissues by subtraction ($J^{Na}_{MS} - J^{Na}_{SM} = J^{Na}_{Net}$). The lines were fitted by least-squares analysis. r^2 = 0.623 and 0.006 for the short-circuit (closed circles) and open-circuit (open circles) conditions, respectively.

We found that there was a positive correlation between these values (r square = 0.62). Taken together, under short-circuit conditions, these results suggest that glucose-induced $\Delta J^{Na}{}_{MS}$ is mainly mediated by SGLT1 and there is less contribution, if any, from other Na^+ transport mechanisms involved in glucose-induced $\Delta J^{Na}{}_{MS}$ increments.

2.3. Activation of SGLT1 does not Increase Mucosal to Serosal $^{22}Na^+$ Fluxes under Open-Circuit Conditions

To mimic physiological conditions, we conducted identical Ussing chamber experiments as in Figure 1 under open-circuit conditions, which allows for the investigation of paracellular ion pathways [21]. The baseline transepithelial potential difference (V_{te}) was measured and G_t was determined from voltage deflections when applying short-current pulse. The baseline V_{te} was −0.9 ± 0.1 mV (n = 3) referenced to the serosal side. For a comparison with short-circuit conditions, equivalent I_{sc} was determined from V_{te} and G_t by applying Ohm's law. Under open-circuit conditions (Table 1, lower rows), baseline and equivalent I_{sc} were not significantly different from those of short-circuit conditions. We next determined whether basal unidirectional $^{22}Na^+$ flux was affected by basal V_{te}. As shown in Table 1, $J^{Na}{}_{MS}$ and $J^{Na}{}_{SM}$ were not significantly different from those of short-circuit conditions, suggesting that baseline V_{te} does not affect basal transcellular and paracellular Na^+ transport. We next measured glucose-induced transepithelial potential difference changes (ΔV_{te}) and ΔJ^{Na} under open-circuit conditions (Figure 3). On the one hand, addition of 10 mM luminal glucose increased the V_{te} (ΔV_{te} −6.3 ± 0.3 mV, n = 6).

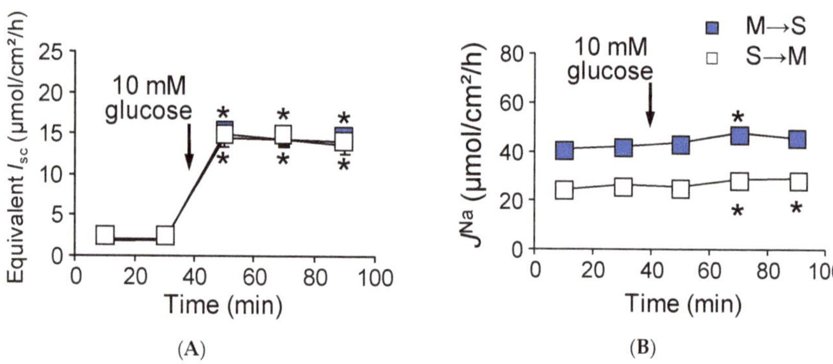

Figure 3. Open-circuit conditions attenuate glucose-induced $J^{Na}{}_{MS}$ in wild-type mice: Glucose-induced equivalent short-circuit current changes (**A**) and $^{22}Na^+$ unidirectional flux changes (J^{Na}) (**B**) were measured simultaneously under open-circuit conditions. Equivalent short-circuit current was determined from transepithelial potential differences and transepithelial conductance by applying Ohm's law as described in the Materials and Methods. Where indicated by the arrows, glucose was added to the mucosal side. Each point represents means ± SE (n = 5 and 5, M to S and S to M, respectively). Where error bars are absent, they are smaller than the symbol used. * $p < 0.05$ as compared with the control.

The equivalent ΔI_{sc} was 12.1 ± 0.8 μmol/cm²/h (Figure 3A), which was not significantly different from that of short-circuit conditions as shown in Figure 1A (p = 0.20). On the other hand, glucose-induced $\Delta J^{Na}{}_{MS}$ increment was significantly inhibited by 60% as compared with that of short-circuit conditions (Figure 3B, $\Delta J^{Na}{}_{MS}$, 4.7 ± 1.2 vs. 12.5 ± 0.8 μmol/cm²/h, p = 0.0001, open-circuit and short-circuit conditions, respectively). Interestingly, the unidirectional serosal to mucosal $^{22}Na^+$ flux was significantly increased after luminal application of glucose (Figure 3B, open squares 25.2 ± 0.9 vs. 28.8 ± 1.4 μmol/cm²/h, p = 0.0003, before and after addition of glucose, respectively), which was not observed under short-circuit conditions (Figure 1B open squares). These results imply that glucose-induced luminal negativity drives the unidirectional serosal to mucosal $^{22}Na^+$ flux via paracellular pathways.

We next assessed the quantitative relationship between ΔI_{sc} and ΔJ^{Na}_{Net} under open-circuit conditions (Figure 2, open circles). There was no relationship between ΔI_{sc} and ΔJ^{Na}_{Net} (r square = 0.006) and the averaged ΔJ^{Na}_{Net} value (1.7 ± 1.3 μmol/cm²/h) was not significantly different from zero ($p = 0.36$). Taken together, these results suggest that Na^+-dependent glucose cotransport does not concomitantly increase transepithelial Na^+ absorption under open-circuit conditions.

2.4. Baseline Na^+ Absorption Mechanisms in Claudin-15 Deficient Mice

To evaluate the impact of deficiency of claudin-15 on Na^+ absorption in the small intestine, we first measured unidirectional $^{22}Na^+$ flux across the jejunum of claudin-15 deficient (*cldn15*$^{-/-}$) mice under short-circuit conditions (Table 2). The J^{Na}_{MS} was decreased by 40% in *cldn15*$^{-/-}$ mice as compared with wild-type mice (31.9 ± 1.9 vs. 51.4 ± 2.3 μmol/cm²/h). In addition, J^{Na}_{SM}, which is mainly reflected by the paracellular pathway, was also decreased by 60% in *cldn15*$^{-/-}$ mice (10.4 ± 0.8 vs. 24.6 ± 1.7 μmol/cm²/h). We also observed a reduced conductance across jejunal preparations from *cldn15*$^{-/-}$ mice (17.7 ± 0.7 vs. 58.7 ± 2.2 mS/cm², $p < 0.0001$ in *cldn15*$^{-/-}$ and wild-type mice, respectively). It has been shown that electrical conductance of the paracellular pathways accounts for 95% of the total conductance in the small intestine [9]. These results suggest that paracellular Na^+-selective pores are mainly formed by claudin-15, consistent with a previous report [14]. The magnitude of the net $^{22}Na^+$ flux was not significantly different than that of wild-type mice (21.4 ± 2.4 vs. 26.9 ± 1.5 μmol/cm²/h, in *cldn15*$^{-/-}$ and wild-type mice, respectively), suggesting that net Na^+ absorption occurs via an electroneutral mechanism. In contrast, the basal I_{sc} was significantly greater than that of wild-type mice (3.3 ± 0.4 vs. 2.4 ± 0.5 μmol/cm²/h, in *cldn15*$^{-/-}$ and wild-type mice, respectively). Therefore, we assessed the contribution of NHE3 to $^{22}Na^+$ unidirectional fluxes under baseline conditions. In the presence of the NHE3 inhibitor S3226, basal J^{Na}_{MS} was inhibited and this magnitude of S3226-sensitive inhibition was similar to that of wild-type mice (Tables 1 and 2, 9.6 vs. 12.5 μmol/cm²/h, in *cldn15*$^{-/-}$ and wild-type mice, respectively). Interestingly, the J^{Na}_{SM} and G_t were significantly decreased by S3226 (Table 2, $p = 0.001$ and 0.018, J^{Na}_{SM} and G_t, respectively), suggesting that paracellular ion permeability was affected by S3226 in *cldn15*$^{-/-}$ but not wild-type mice. However, we did not further explore this mechanism in this study. Jointly, these results suggest that although other NHE isoforms may be involved in electroneutral Na^+ absorption, basal net Na^+ absorption is mostly dependent on NHE3 transport, similar to wild-type mice. In addition, paracellular Na^+-selective pores, which are formed mainly by claudin-15, were decreased in *cldn15*$^{-/-}$ mice.

Table 2. Basal $^{22}Na^+$ flux and electrical parameters in *cldn15*$^{-/-}$ mice.

	J^{Na}, μmol/cm²/h			I_{sc}, μmol/cm²/h	G_t, mS/cm²	n
	M→S	S→M	Net			
			Short-Circuit Conditions			
Control	31.9 ± 1.9 †	10.4 ± 0.8 †	21.4 ± 2.4	3.3 ± 0.4 †	17.7 ± 0.7 †	6
S3226	22.3 ± 1.5 *	5.8 ± 0.5 *	16.4 ± 1.0	3.9 ± 0.1	13.6 ± 1.0 *	4
			Open-Circuit Conditions			
Control	35.6 ± 2.4 N.S.	12.0 ± 0.9 N.S.	23.7 ± 2.4	4.0 ± 0.6	19.4 ± 1.4	6

10 μM S3226 was added to the mucosal side. Each value represents the mean ± SE. * $p < 0.05$ as compared with the control. N.S. not significant as compared with short-circuit conditions. † $p < 0.05$ as compared with the same conditions in wild-type mice as shown in Table 1. M→S indicates the unidirectional mucosal to serosal Na^+ flux. S→M indicates the unidirectional serosal to mucosal Na^+ flux. n: Number of animals examined.

2.5. Na^+-Dependent Glucose Transporter SGLT1 Is Up-Regulated in *Cldn15*$^{-/-}$ Mice

We first confirmed the expression of claudin-15 by immunofluorescence (Figure 4A) and quantitative RT-PCR (Figure 4B) experiments in the duodenum and jejunum. In wild-type mice, claudin-15 colocalized with another tight junction protein occludin. However, claudin-15 signals were completely abolished in *cldn15*$^{-/-}$ mice, consistent with a previous study [13]. It has been shown that glucose malabsorption occurs in *cldn15*$^{-/-}$ mice [14]. To elucidate the mechanism underlining these impairments, I_{sc} was measured in *cldn15*$^{-/-}$ mice. The addition of glucose to the mucosal side increased the I_{sc} in a dose-dependent manner (Figure 4C). This change in I_{sc} conformed to Michaelis–Menten kinetics (Figure 4D, r square = 0.996 ± 0.0001, n = 6), and the value of the maximum change in I_{sc} (V_{max}) was three-fold increased (p = 0.034 by the Mann–Whitney test 1479 ± 426 vs. 426 ± 51 μA/cm^2/h in *cldn15*$^{-/-}$ and wild-type mice, respectively).

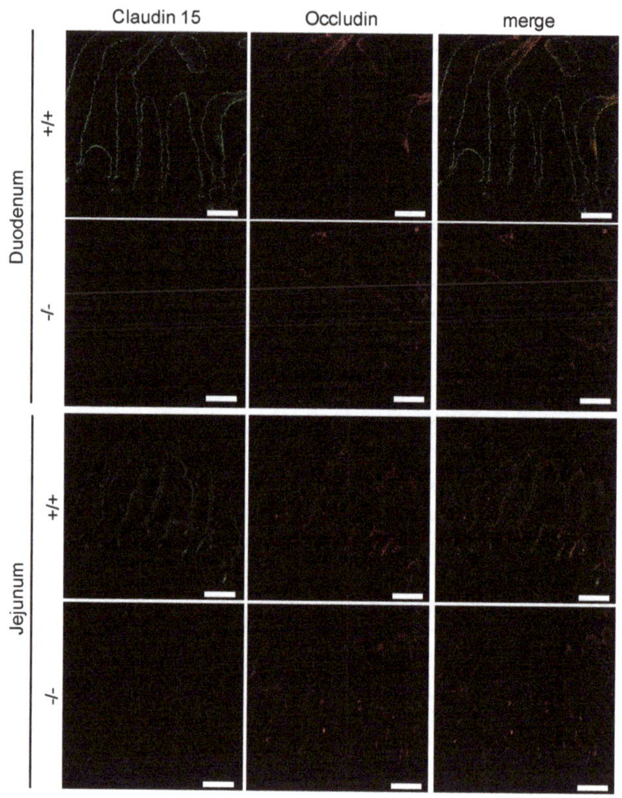

(A)

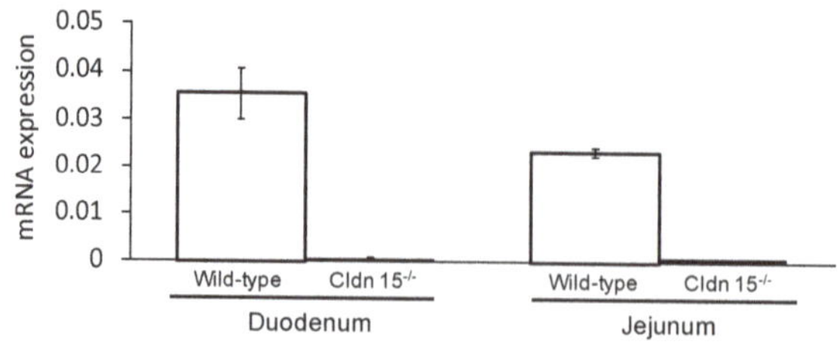

(B)

Figure 4. *Cont.*

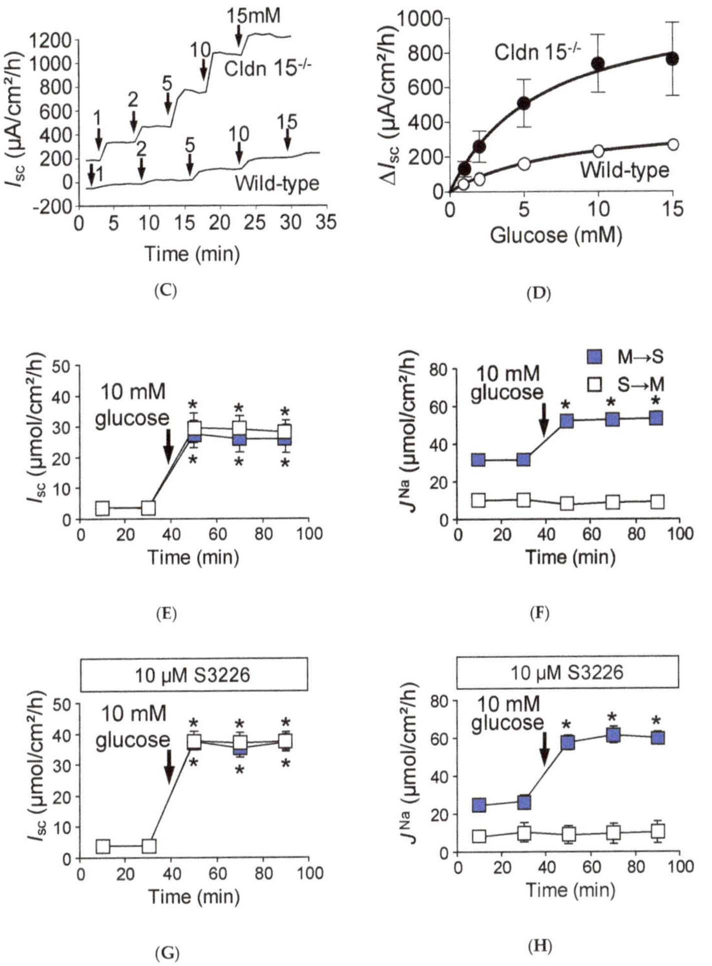

Figure 4. Representative confocal images of double immunofluorescence staining of claudin-15 (green) and occluding (red) (**A**) (n = 3) and quantitative RT-PCR (**B**) (n = 3) in wild-type and *cldn15*$^{-/-}$ mice. Bar, 100 μm. Activation of SGLT1 increases glucose-induced $J^{Na}{}_{MS}$ under short-circuit conditions in *cldn15*$^{-/-}$ mice: Representative I_{sc} trace of glucose-induced I_{sc} changes in *cldn15*$^{-/-}$ and wild-type mice (**C**), where, indicated by the arrows, glucose was added to the mucosal side, the final concentration of glucose is shown in mM; and the concentration dependence of the glucose-induced I_{sc} (**D**). The curve was fit to the Michaelis–Menten equation (n = 3 and 6, wild-type, and *cldn15*$^{-/-}$ mice, respectively). Where error bars are absent, they are smaller than the symbol used. The 10 mM glucose-induced short-circuit current changes (I_{sc}) (**E**) and $^{22}Na^+$ unidirectional flux changes (J^{Na}) (**F**) were measured simultaneously the same as Figure 1 (n = 7 and 7, M to S and S to M, respectively). Where indicated by the arrows, glucose was added to the mucosal side. The effect of S3226 on glucose-induced ΔI_{sc} (**G**) and ΔJ^{Na} (**H**) (n = 5 and 5, M to S and S to M, respectively). Where indicated by the arrows, glucose was added to the mucosal side. Each point represents the mean ± SE. Where error bars are absent, they are smaller than the symbol used. * $p < 0.05$ as compared with the baseline control.

However, the Michaelis–Menten constant (K_m) was not significantly different than that of wild-type mice ($p = 0.23$ by the Mann–Whitney test, 11.4 ± 2.0 vs. 8.4 ± 2.0 mM in *cldn15*$^{-/-}$ and wild-type mice, respectively). Together, these results imply that the total number of SGLT1 transporters was increased in *cldn15*$^{-/-}$ mice to compensate for the lowered luminal Na^+ concentration [22].

The addition of 10 mM glucose to the mucosal side resulted in an increase of I_{sc} (Figure 4E, ΔI_{sc}: 23.9 ± 3.8 μmol/cm^2/h) and $J^{Na}{}_{MS}$ (Figure 4F closed squares, 21.4 ± 2.4 μmol/cm^2/h), while serosal to mucosal $J^{Na}{}_{SM}$ was not significantly changed after addition of luminal glucose (Figure 4F open squares, 10.0 ± 0.8 vs. 8.7 ± 0.5 μmol/cm^2/h, p = 0.053, before and after addition of glucose, respectively). Since luminal Na^+ homeostasis was disturbed in *cldn15*$^{-/-}$ mice [22], we next assessed the contribution of luminal Na^+/H^+ exchanger NHE3 to glucose-induced $J^{Na}{}_{MS}$ increments by using the NHE3 specific inhibitor S3226. The addition of glucose to the mucosal side resulted in an increase of I_{sc} (Figure 4G ΔI_{sc}: 33.6 ± 2.5 μmol/cm^2/h), which is slightly higher in the absence of S3226 (p = 0.003). In the presence of S3226, glucose-induced $J^{Na}{}_{MS}$ increment was also observed (Figure 4H closed squares, $\Delta J^{Na}{}_{MS}$: 34.9 ± 2.2 μmol/cm^2/h), suggesting that NHE3 is not responsible for glucose-induced $^{22}Na^+$ unidirectional flux increments. We next assessed the quantitative relationship between ΔI_{sc} and $\Delta J^{Na}{}_{Net}$ (Figure 5, closed circles). There was a positive correlation between ΔI_{sc} and $\Delta J^{Na}{}_{Net}$ (r square = 0.67). Taken together, these results suggest that glucose-induced $\Delta J^{Na}{}_{MS}$ is mainly mediated by SGLT1 under short-circuit conditions in *cldn15*$^{-/-}$ mice, which is the same as in wild-type mice.

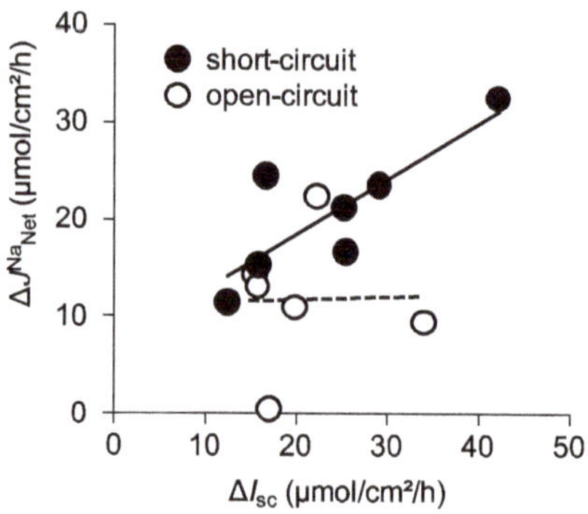

Figure 5. The relationship between changes of glucose-induced I_{sc} and changes of glucose-induced net $^{22}Na^+$ fluxes in *cldn15*$^{-/-}$ mice: Glucose-induced ΔI_{sc} and $J^{Na}{}_{Net}$ were calculated from the data of Figures 4 and 6 and replotted the same as in Figure 2. The lines were fitted by least-squares analysis. r^2 = 0.67 and 0.0012 for the short-circuit and open-circuit conditions, respectively.

2.6. *Absence of Claudin-15 Increases Glucose-Induced Mucosal to Serosal $^{22}Na^+$ Flux*

We next measured basal electrical parameters and $^{22}Na^+$ flux under open-circuit conditions in *cldn15*$^{-/-}$ mice (Table 2, lower rows). Baseline V_{te} was −6.0 ± 1.2 mV referenced to the serosal side (equivalent I_{sc} 4.0 ± 0.6 μmol/cm^2/h). Under those conditions, we examined whether basal unidirectional $^{22}Na^+$ flux was affected by V_{te}. Although there was a negative luminal V_{te}, which is preferential for increasing serosal to mucosal Na^+ flux, the $J^{Na}{}_{SM}$ was not significantly different from those of short-circuit conditions (10.4 ± 0.8 vs. 12.0 ± 0.9 in short- and open-circuit conditions, respectively). We next measured glucose-induced V_{te} and J^{Na} under open-circuit conditions (Figure 6). The addition of 10 mM luminal glucose increased the V_{te} (ΔV_{te} −20.6 ± 2.9 mV), which corresponded to an equivalent ΔI_{sc} (24.7 ± 2.5 μmol/cm^2/h, Figure 6A). This equivalent ΔI_{sc} was not significantly different from that of short-circuit conditions, as shown in Figure 4C (p = 0.32). Unlike wild-type mice, there was a large negative luminal V_{te}, and a robust glucose-induced mucosal to serosal $^{22}Na^+$ flux increment was observed in *cldn15*$^{-/-}$ mice (14.5 ± 1.9 vs. 4.7 ± 1.2 mmol/cm^2/h, p = 0.01, in *cldn15*$^{-/-}$ and wild-type mice, respectively, Figure 6B). After application of glucose, an increase of $J^{Na}{}_{SM}$ would be expected from such a large negative luminal V_{te}, however, $J^{Na}{}_{SM}$ did not significantly change (Figure 6B, open squares). These results suggest that paracellular Na^+ permeability was decreased in *cldn15*$^{-/-}$ mice. We next assessed the quantitative relationship between ΔI_{sc} and $\Delta J^{Na}{}_{Net}$ under open-circuit conditions (Figure 5, open circles). There was no relationship between ΔI_{sc} and $\Delta J^{Na}{}_{Net}$ (r square = 0.0012). However, the averaged $\Delta J^{Na}{}_{Net}$ value (11.5 ± 2.9 μmol/cm^2/h) was significantly different from zero (p = 0.01). Taken together, these results suggest that Na^+-dependent glucose cotransport concomitantly increases transepithelial Na^+ transport under open-circuit conditions in *cldn15*$^{-/-}$ mice.

To quantitatively evaluate the V_{te}-dependent paracellular passive Na^+ flux, we examined the effect of changing V_{te} on $J^{Na}{}_{SM}$, which mainly represents the paracellular pathway. $J^{Na}{}_{SM}$ was plotted as a function of (FΔV/RT)/{exp(FΔV/RT) − 1}, which represents the driving force of ion movement. This should yield a line having a slope of the V_{te}-dependent diffusion flux [23]. As shown in Figure 7, the slope of the line was decreased by 50% in *cldn15*$^{-/-}$ mice as compared with wild-type mice (3.6 ± 0.9 vs. 7.8 ± 1.9, in *cldn15*$^{-/-}$ and wild-type mice, respectively), suggesting decreased paracellular Na^+ permeability in *cldn15*$^{-/-}$ mice. Together, these results suggest that the Na^+ which is absorbed by Na^+-dependent glucose cotransport is recycled back into the lumen to support Na^+-dependent glucose absorption and this Na^+-cotransport induced luminal negative potential is important for Na^+ recycling in wild-type mice.

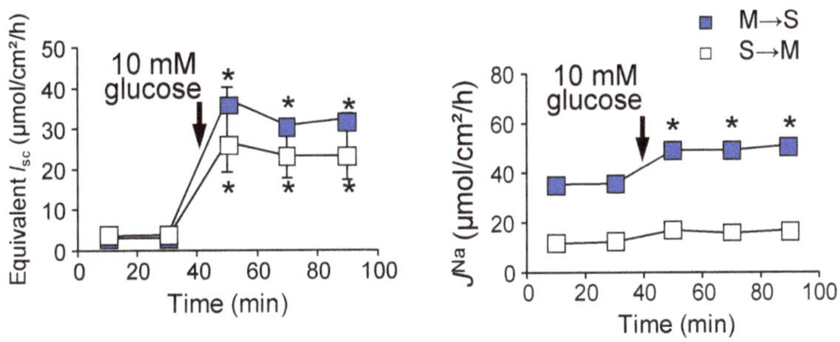

(A) (B)

Figure 6. Robust glucose-induced $J^{Na}{}_{MS}$ are observed in *cldn15*$^{-/-}$ mice under open-circuit conditions: Glucose-induced equivalent I_{sc} (**A**) and ΔJ^{Na} (**B**) were measured simultaneously under open-circuit conditions. Where indicated by the arrows, glucose was added to the mucosal side. Equivalent I_{sc} was determined the same as in Figure 3. Closed squares indicate $J^{Na}{}_{MS}$ and open squares indicate $J^{Na}{}_{SM}$ (n = 7 and 6, M to S and S to M, respectively). Each point represents the mean ± SE. Where error bars are absent, they are smaller than the symbol used. * $p < 0.05$ as compared with the baseline control.

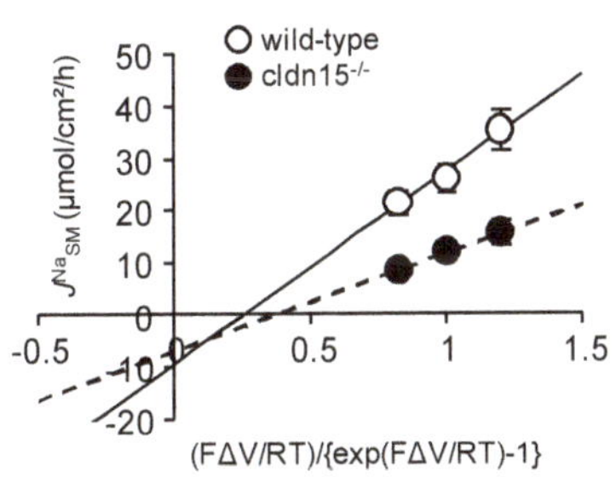

Figure 7. The effect of changing the transepithelial potential on $J^{Na}{}_{SM}$: $J^{Na}{}_{SM}$ was measured at V_{te} = 0 and ± 10 mV. $J^{Na}{}_{SM}$ was plotted as a function of (FΔV$_{te}$/RT)/{exp(FΔV$_{te}$/RT)−1}, where F is the Faraday constant, R is the molar gas constant, and T is the temperature. Lines are fitted with least-squares method. Wild-type (open circles, n = 6) and *cldn15*$^{-/-}$ mice (closed circles, n = 4).

2.7. The Efficiency of Na^+ Recycling Systems Is Reduced in a Cholera Toxin-Induced Diarrhea Model

The preceding experiments suggest that, under physiological conditions, the Na^+ that is absorbed by Na^+-dependent glucose cotransport is recycled back into the lumen via paracellular Na^+ conductance which is driven by the Na^+ cotransport induced luminal negative potential. However, this idea is not consistent with the mechanisms of oral rehydration therapy, which is based on the notion that the Na^+ which is absorbed by Na^+-glucose cotransport enters the systemic circulation [16]. This discrepancy could be explained by the idea that the efficiency of Na^+ recycling systems is reduced during infectious diarrhea. To address this directly, we measured glucose-induced unidirectional $J^{Na}{}_{MS}$ in cholera toxin-diarrhea model mice. Five hours after gavage of cholera toxin, we first verified the effect of cholera toxin on intestinal ion transport by measuring the transepithelial potential difference (V_{te}) in isolated upper small intestine in Ussing chambers. Luminal negative V_{te} (referenced to the serosal side) was increased after administration of cholera toxin (–0.30 ± 0.3 vs. –2.66 ± 0.3 mV in the control and cholera toxin-diarrhea model mice, respectively, $p = 0.008$), suggesting that Cl^- secretion was increased in cholera toxin-diarrhea model mice. In addition, basal unidirectional $J^{Na}{}_{MS}$ was decreased by 42% as compared with the control mice (Table 3) but not for $J^{Na}{}_{SM}$, suggesting inhibition of electroneutral NaCl absorption. These observations are consistent with the action of cholera toxin on intestinal epithelial transport [24]. Interestingly, the basal G_t of cholera toxin-diarrhea model mice was significantly decreased by 27.8% as compared with the control mice (Table 3). Surprisingly, although there was such a large luminal negative V_{te} (2.7 mV), in which an increase of $J^{Na}{}_{SM}$ would be expected as shown in Figure 7, $J^{Na}{}_{SM}$ was actually decreased by 6.2% as compared with the control mice (Table 3). Taken together, these results suggest that paracellular Na^+ pores, which can be formed by claudin-15, are decreased in cholera toxin-diarrhea model mice, consistent with a previous study [25]. To address this question directly, we measured G_t after stimulation of cAMP formation by forskolin and the phosphodiesterase inhibitor isobutylmethylxanthine (IBMX) in wild-type and *cldn15*$^{-/-}$ mice in Ussing chambers. G_t was decreased within 20 min after addition of forskolin and IBMX in wild-type mice (29.1 ± 1.3 vs. 21.8 ± 1.4 mS/cm^2 before and after treatment with forskolin and IBMX, respectively, $p = 0.0001$), consistent with a previous study [26]. However, upon formation of intracellular cAMP induced by forskolin and IBMX, G_t was not decreased in *cldn15*$^{-/-}$ mice (18.6 ± 5.3 vs. 16.5 ± 5.4 mS/cm^2, after treatment with forskolin and IBMX and control, respectively, $p = 0.10$). These results suggest that paracellular Na^+ conductance, which is directed by claudin-15, is acutely regulated by elevation of intracellular cAMP.

Table 3. Basal $^{22}Na^+$ flux and electrical parameters in cholera toxin-diarrhea model.

	J^{Na}, μmol/cm²/h			I_{sc}, μmol/cm²/h	G_t, mS/cm²	n
	M→S	S→M	Net			
	Open-Circuit Conditions					
Control	29.2 ± 2.1	18.4 ± 3.6	10.8 ± 2.8	−1.0 ± 0.2	61.6 ± 9.3	3
Cholera	16.9 ± 1.4 *	17.3 ± 1.4	−0.3 ± 1.0 *	3.9± 0.3 *	39.6 ± 1.1 *	5

Mice were gavaged without (control) or with 10 μg cholera toxin in 150 mM NaCl solution. Five hours after administration, the upper small intestine was excised and used for the Ussing chamber experiments. Each value represents the mean ± SE. * $p < 0.05$ as compared with the control by the Mann–Whitney test. M→S indicates the unidirectional mucosal to serosal Na^+ flux. S→M indicates the unidirectional serosal to mucosal Na^+ flux. n: Number of animals examined.

We next measured glucose-induced mucosal to serosal $^{22}Na^+$ flux in the cholera toxin-diarrhea model mice under open-circuit conditions (Figure 8). The addition of glucose to the mucosal side resulted in an increase in V_{te} (Figure 8A closed squares, ΔV_{te} −2.1 ± 0.3 mV, $n = 5$). As shown in Figure 8B, glucose-induced equivalent ΔI_{sc} was 6.7 ± 1.9 μmol/cm²/h, which was not significantly different from that of control conditions, as shown in Figure 3A ($p = 0.16$). Interestingly, after the addition of glucose, G_t was increased in the cholera toxin-diarrhea model mice, but not in the control mice (Figure 8C). Unlike animals that were not treated with cholera toxin treated with vehicle only (Figure 8D, open squares), robust glucose-induced mucosal to serosal $^{22}Na^+$ flux increment was observed in the cholera toxin-diarrhea model mice (Figure 8D, 11.1 ± 1.8 vs. 6.1 ± 1.6 μmol/cm²/h, $p = 0.08$ as compared with the control conditions, in the cholera toxin-diarrhea model and the control mice, respectively). It failed to attain statistical significance, but the phenomenon is reminiscent of the *cldn15*$^{-/-}$ mice (Figure 6B). Taken together, these results suggest that the efficiency of Na^+ recycling systems is reduced under cholera toxin diarrhea conditions.

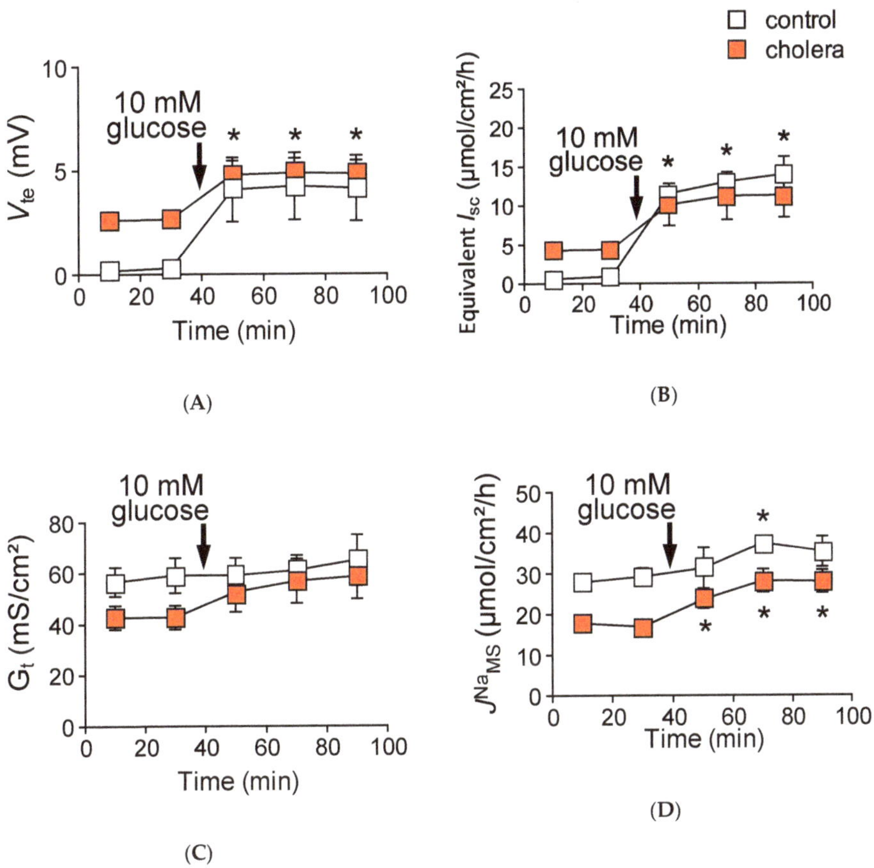

Figure 8. Robust glucose-induced J^{Na}_{MS} is observed in cholera toxin-diarrhea model mice under open-circuit conditions: Glucose-induced V_{te} (**A**), equivalent I_{sc} (**B**), and ΔJ^{Na} (**D**) were measured simultaneously under open-circuit conditions. Equivalent I_{sc} was determined the same as in Figure 3. G_t (**C**) was determined from transepithelial potential difference (V_{te}) and current pulse by applying Ohm's law. Open squares indicate control conditions (without cholera toxin) and closed squares indicate cholera toxin treated conditions ($n = 3$ and 5, control and cholera toxin treated mice, respectively). Where indicated by the arrows, glucose was added to the mucosal side. Each point represents the mean ± SE. Where error bars are absent, they are smaller than the symbol used. * $p < 0.05$ as compared with the baseline control.

3. Discussion

The aim of this study was to investigate if paracellular recirculation of Na^+ is essential to support Na^+-dependent nutrient absorption and to elucidate the role of Na^+-nutrient cotransport induced luminal negative potential for Na^+ recycling. We demonstrated that under short-circuit conditions luminal application of glucose resulted in an increment of absorptive $^{22}Na^+$ fluxes (ΔJ^{Na}) which corresponded to increments of short-circuit currents (ΔI_{sc}) in wild-type mice. However, under open-circuit conditions, ΔI_{sc} was observed but ΔJ^{Na} was strongly inhibited. In *cldn15*$^{-/-}$ mice, a robust increment of ΔJ^{Na} was observed under open-circuit conditions, and this recycling dysfunction was mimicked by a cholera toxin-diarrhea model in wild-type mice. Therefore, we feel that under physiological conditions, the Na^+ that is absorbed with nutrients is recycled back into the lumen via the paracellular pathway due to pores which are formed by claudin-15. To further support this idea, the efficiency of this Na^+ recycling system was also reduced in cholera toxin-diarrhea model mice.

3.1. Intestinal Nutrient Absorption Mechanisms Need a Large Amount of Luminal Na^+

We assumed that most protein and carbohydrates are digested to monomers and absorbed via Na^+-dependent nutrient transporters. However, it has been proposed that a significant amount of amino acids are absorbed as tripeptides by transporters driven by protons [27]. We have previously shown that the mucosal surface pH in the upper jejunum is significantly alkalinized and glycyl-sarcosine (nonhydrolyzable dipeptide, Gly-Sar) absorption was inhibited in *cldn15*$^{-/-}$ mice [22]. Furthermore, Gly-Sar induced I_{sc} increments were tightly coupled to luminal Na^+/H^+ exchange NHE3 activity and these peptide-induced I_{sc} increments were inhibited by NHE3 specific inhibitors S3226 and Tenapanor [22,28]. These results imply that other proton dependent cotransporters systems such as proton coupled amino acid and peptide transporters need luminal Na^+. With respect to carbohydrates, it has been shown that complex carbohydrates can reduce the influx of carbohydrates monomers [29], which suggests that our estimation that most carbohydrates are digested to monomers is oversimplified. However, this is unlikely based on the observation that small intestinal mass absorption of glucose is mainly mediated by SGLT1, since the increase of glucose concentration in plasma after glucose gavage is reduced in SGLT1 knock-out mice [30]. Taken together, these considerations suggest that intestinal nutrient absorption mechanisms require a large amount of luminal Na^+.

3.2. Paracellular Na^+ Permeability Is Decreased in Cldn15$^{-/-}$ Mice

It has been shown that small intestinal epithelia are classified as leaky epithelia, i.e., paracellular conductance greater than ~90% of total tissue conductance and cation selective permselectivity ($P_{Na} > P_{Cl}$) [9]. However, the molecules responsible for permselectivity in the intestine remain to be fully elucidated. We found that electrical transepithelial conductance of *cldn15*$^{-/-}$ mice was decreased by 70% as compared with wild-type mice (Tables 1 and 2). In addition, unidirectional $^{22}Na^+$ flux from serosal to mucosal side in *cldn15*$^{-/-}$ mice, which is mainly reflected by the paracellular pathway, was decreased by 60% as compared with wild-type mice (Figures 4F and 1B). Taken together, these results suggest that paracellular Na^+ pores are mainly formed by claudin-15, consistent with a previous report [14]. Despite having defective luminal Na^+ homeostasis [22], *cldn15*$^{-/-}$ mice do not have severe intestinal dysfunction and malabsorption (serum albumin 2.7 ± 0.19 vs. 3.0 ± 0.12g/dL, $p = 0.17$; serum total glyceride 43 ± 13 vs. 47 ± 20 mg/dL, $p = 0.88$; serum glucose 205 ± 10 vs. 270 ± 27 mg/dL, $p = 0.1$ in *cldn15*$^{-/-}$ and wild-type mice, respectively, $n = 3$ to 4 in each genotype). We believe this can be explained by the other remaining claudin(s), which could be sufficient to support the luminal Na^+ which is needed for nutrient absorption. One possibility is that claudin-2, which forms cation-selective pores, can contribute to Na^+ dependent nutrient absorption [11,31]. Indeed, it has been shown that claudin-2 and claudin-15 double-knockout mice die as a result of malnutrition in early infancy [32], suggesting that claudin-2 could also be contributing to Na^+-dependent nutrient absorption.

3.3. Luminal Negative Potential Is Important for Na^+ Recirculation

Our data support the conclusion that Na^+ absorbed by Na^+-dependent glucose cotransport is rapidly recycled back into the lumen via paracellular pathways which are driven by increased luminal negative potential generated by electrogenic glucose absorption mechanisms. Under open-circuit conditions, activation of SGLT1 did not increase mucosal to serosal $^{22}Na^+$ fluxes in wild-type mice (Figure 3B). Furthermore, under the same experimental conditions, although there was a large luminal negative V_{te} (−20 mV), robust glucose-induced mucosal to serosal $^{22}Na^+$ flux increment was observed in *cldn15*$^{-/-}$ mice (Figure 6B). To our knowledge, under physiological conditions, a postprandial robust increase in blood Na^+ concentrations has not been shown. However, it is generally believed that there are two Na^+ absorption systems in the small intestine; one is electrogenic nutrient-coupled Na^+ absorption, and the other is electroneutral NaCl absorption [1]. It is also generally thought that bulk transport of NaCl absorption in the small intestine is mediated by electroneutral absorption by the coupling of luminal Na^+/H^+ exchanger NHE3, and Cl^-/HCO_3^- exchanger SLC26A3, since both NHE3 knockout mice and SLC26A3 knockout mice manifest in diarrhea [33,34]. These two sets of Na^+ absorption transporter systems reside in the same nutrient absorbing enterocytes. It is predicted, therefore, that there is an interaction between the two Na^+ absorption mechanisms. Indeed, it has been shown that Na^+-coupled glucose uptake stimulates NHE3 transport activity in mouse jejunum [19]. However, this interaction would not be favorable for the driving force of nutrient-coupled Na^+ absorption because a decrease of luminal Na^+ concentration is not favorable for Na^+-dependent nutrient absorption to absorb nutrients efficiently. Our results indicated that glucose does not stimulate NHE3 activity (Figure 1D). In addition, we fed rats with nominal Na-free diet for five days and measured intestinal luminal Na^+ concentration. There was a significant difference in luminal Na^+ concentrations in the stomach (59 ± 9 vs. 7 ± 1 mM in control and Na-free diet, respectively, $p < 0.05$) and colon (40 ± 8 vs. 18 ± 4 mM in control and Na-free diet, respectively, $p < 0.05$) but not in in the small intestine (57 ± 13 vs. 50 ± 9 mM in control and Na-free diet, respectively, $p > 0.05$). These results suggest that luminal Na^+ homeostasis in the small intestine, which is the external milieu, is independent of the amount of Na^+ intake. We believe that this luminal Na^+ homeostasis is maintained by claudin-15 and regulated by increased luminal potential generated by electrogenic Na^+-nutrient cotransport, since luminal Na^+ homeostasis is disrupted in *cldn15*$^{-/-}$ mice [22]. Under pathophysiological conditions in wild-type mice, our results indicated that paracellular Na^+ conductance was decreased by cholera toxin (Table 3). In accordance, previous studies have shown that paracellular conductance and ion selectivity were changed after treatment with theophylline (phosphodiesterase inhibitor, which raises intracellular cAMP) or cholera toxin in the rabbit ileum [25]. It has also been shown that an increase of intracellular cAMP resulted in a decrease of paracellular conductance [26,35]. Our results imply that Na^+ conductance that is directed by claudin-15 is regulated by intracellular cAMP level. However, elucidation of molecular mechanism of this regulation requires further investigation.

3.4. Physiological Relevance of the Na^+ Recirculation System in the Small Intestine

On the one hand, our conclusion implies that the Na^+ that is absorbed by SGLT1 does not enter the systemic circulation under physiological conditions (Figure 9A). On the other hand, under pathophysiological conditions, such as in cholera-infected patients, glucose-containing oral rehydration solution (ORS) stimulates Na^+ and water absorption, implying that the Na^+ that is absorbed by SGLT1 does enter the systemic circulation (Figure 9B). It is also thought that glucose-induced Na^+ absorption is not affected by cholera toxin [36]. The composition (75 mM glucose, 75 mM NaCl, and so on) of ORS is based on its efficacy in replacing water and electrolytes in individuals [16,37]. This glucose-dependent Na^+-absorption mechanism under pathophysiological conditions is not consistent with our results under normal conditions, where Na^+ absorbed with glucose is recycled back into the lumen rather than entering systemic circulation. Another explanation for glucose-induced Na^+ absorption could be a decrease of Na^+ recirculation upon infection with cholera. Indeed, our findings indicated that paracellular Na^+ pores were decreased and glucose-induced Na^+ absorption was observed in cholera toxin-diarrhea model mice under open-circuit conditions (Figure 8). These findings are consistent with the notion that Na^+ recycling systems were reduced under pathophysiological diarrhea conditions. Our findings also suggest that Na^+ cotransport-induced luminal negative potential is important for the Na^+ recycling system. Conversely, this implies that Na^+ absorbed via electroneutral systems, such as

NaCl absorption (parallelly coupled Na^+/H^+ and Cl^-/HCO_3^- exchangers) and nonelectrogenic fructose absorption, can enter systemic circulation. In accordance with this notion, a recent study demonstrated that fructose-induced hypertension is initiated by increased absorption of NaCl and fructose in the intestine [38]. It is also noteworthy that ORS was occasionally associated with hypernatremia [39], implying that there is a decrease of Na^+ recycling system activity in cases of infectious diarrhea (Figure 9B).

In summary, our data indicate that claudin-15 is important for luminal Na^+ homeostasis and Na^+-dependent nutrient absorption. These findings may contribute to the understanding of the mechanisms of oral rehydration therapy. Our observations raise the possibility that the Na^+ that is absorbed with nutrients is recycled back into the lumen via paracellular pores which are formed mainly by claudin-15 under physiological conditions.

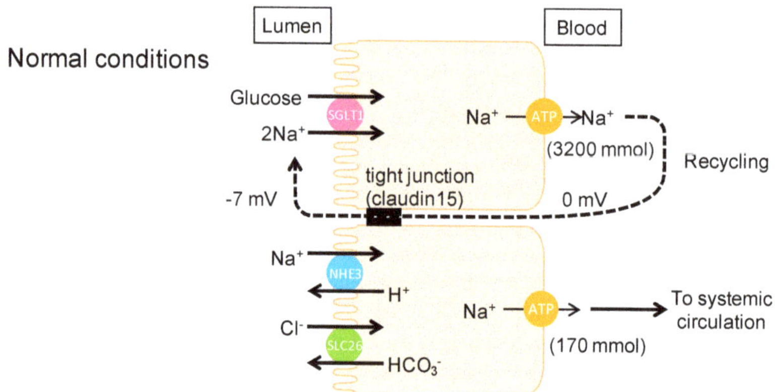

(**A**)

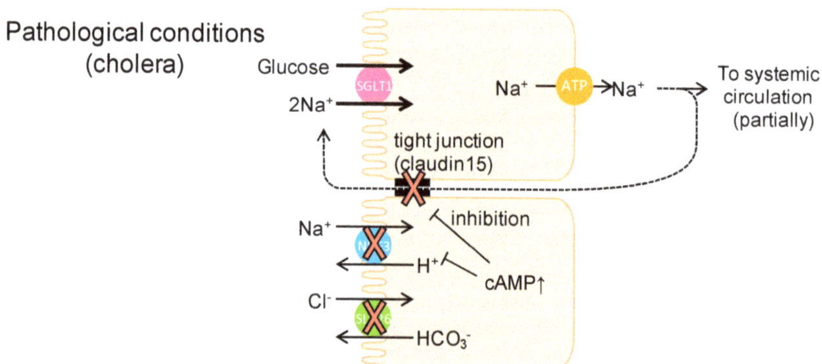

(**B**)

Figure 9. Schematic illustration of Na^+ recycling mechanisms in the murine small intestine: Under normal physiological conditions (**A**), Na^+, which is absorbed with glucose, is recycled back into the lumen. However, under pathological conditions (**B**), the Na^+ that is absorbed with glucose can be partially transported to systemic circulation. Dashed lines indicate the Na^+ recirculation and the thickness of lines indicate the amount of Na^+. T-bars indicate inhibition. For more detail, see Discussion.

4. Materials and Methods

4.1. Ethical Approval

All animal experimental procedures and handling were approved by the Animal Care and Use Committee of the University of Shizuoka (reference no.165117 and 175151, approved on 28th March 2016 and 8th March 2017, respectively) and conducted in accordance with the Guidelines and Regulations for the Care and Use of Experimental Animals by the University of Shizuoka.

4.2. Animals

Claudin-15 deficient (*Cldn15*$^{-/-}$) mice were originally generated in the Laboratory of Prof. Tsukita, as described previously [13]. *Cldn15*$^{-/-}$ mice on a C57BL/6J genetic background and their age- and sex-matched wild-type mice were used. Wild-type male C57BL/6J Jcl mice from Clea Japan (Tokyo, Japan) were also used in some experiments. Mice were used at 2 to 9 months of age. The mice were fed a standard pellet diet (MF, Oriental Yeast, Tokyo, Japan), and water was provided ad libitum.

4.3. Measurement of Electrical Parameters and Unidirectional Fluxes of $^{22}Na^+$ and $^{36}Cl^-$

Mice were anaesthetized with a mixture of drugs (10 μL/g B.W., I.P. injection) consisting of medetomidine (30 μg/mL, Nippon Zenyaku Kogyo, Fukushima, Japan), midazolam (0.4 mg/mL, Teva Pharma Ltd., Nagoya, Japan), and butorphanol (0.5 mg/mL, Meiji Seika, Tokyo, Japan). The abdomen was opened by a midline incision, the small intestine from duodenum to terminal ileum was excised, and the middle one-third of the small intestine was used for experiments. The isolated segment was opened and rinsed with ice-cold oxygenized buffer to remove luminal contents, and then the muscle layer was stripped with fine forceps under a stereomicroscope. The tissue was then mounted vertically in Ussing chambers with an internal surface area of 0.2 cm^2. The bathing solution in each chamber was 5 mL and was kept at 37 °C in a water-jacketed reservoir. The bathing solution contained (in mM) 119 NaCl, 21 $NaHCO_3$, 2.4 K_2HPO_4, 0.6 KH_2PO_4, 1.2 $CaCl_2$, 1.2 $MgCl_2$, 0.5 glutamine, and 10 μM indomethacin, and was gassed with 95% O_2 and 5% CO_2 (pH 7.4). I_{sc} was recorded using a voltage-clamping amplifier (CEZ9100, Nihon Kohden, Tokyo, Japan). G_t was calculated from the change of current in response to voltage pulses according to Ohm's law. We also performed experiments under open-circuit conditions to compare electrophysiological parameters and ion flux with those under short-circuited conditions. The equivalent I_{sc} was determined from V_{te} and G_t by applying Ohm's law. The unidirectional transmural radioactive isotope fluxes of mucosal to serosal (J_{MS}) and serosal to mucosal (J_{SM}) were measured in adjacent tissues. Then, 9 kBq/mL $^{22}Na^+$ or 1.6 kBq/mL $^{36}Cl^-$ was added either to the serosal or mucosal solutions after reaching stable electrical parameters. After a 45 min period of equilibration, samples (0.5 mL each) were taken from the unlabeled side at 20 min intervals and replaced with an equal volume of unlabeled solution. Medium samples containing $^{22}Na^+$ and $^{36}Cl^-$ were counted in a liquid scintillation counter (LSC-7000, Aloka, Tokyo, Japan). To examine the effect of V_{te} change on unidirectional $^{22}Na^+$ flux, we performed two 20 min flux periods with V_{te} at 0 mV, and two 20 min periods with V_{te} at 10 mV (or −10 mV).

4.4. Cholera Toxin-Induced Diarrhea Model

Before the administration of cholera toxin (Wako, Osaka, Japan), mice were fasted for 24 h except for water ingestion. Mice were then gavaged with a single dose of 10 μg cholera toxin in 100 μL of 150 mM NaCl solution through a gastric tube, with NaCl solution as a control. Five hours after administration, mice were anaesthetized with a mixture of drugs, the duodenum and upper part of jejunum were excised and used for the Ussing chamber experiments.

4.5. Chemicals

3-[2-(3-guanidino-2-methyl-3-oxopropenyl)-5-methyl-phenyl]-N-isopropylidene-2-methyl-acrylamide dihydrochloride (S3226) was synthesized by WuXi AppTec Co., Ltd. (Shanghai, People's Republic of China). The S3226 was dissolved in 0.1% DMSO to make stock solutions. The $^{36}Cl^-$ was purchased from Amersham Bioscience (Piscataway, NJ, USA), $^{22}Na^+$ was purchased from Perkin-Elmer (Boston, MA, USA) and all other reagents were from Sigma (St. Louis, MO, USA).

4.6. Real-Time Quantitative PCR

Real-time quantitative PCR experiments were performed as previously described in [22]. The following primers were used for PCR amplifications: *Cldn15*, 5′-CAACGTGGCAACATGGA-3′ and 5′-TGACGGCGTACCACGAGATAG-3′; *beta-actin*, 5′-CATCCGTAAAGACCTCTATGCCAAC-3′ and 5′-ATGGAGCCACCGATCCACA-3′.

4.7. Immunofluorescence

The small intestine was excised as in the flux experiments and opened and rinsed with ice cold PBS. The tissue segment was coated with Tissue-Tek® OCT compound (Sakura Finetek, Tokyo, Japan), and embedded into a mold containing OCT compound and frozen at −80 °C. Frozen specimens were cut in 5 µm slices using a Cryostat (CM3050 S; Leica Biosystems, Nussloch, Germany) and put on coverslips. Sections were dried for 30 min, and, then, incubated in 95% ethanol on ice for 30 min. Coverslips were then bathed in acetone for one minute and rinsed 3 times in PBS. The tissue was preblocked with 5% skim milk powder in 0.1% Triton X®-100 in PBS (0.1% PBST) for 30 min. The coverslips were incubated with primary antibodies for claudin-15 or occludin (kindly gifted from Prof. M. Furuse, National Institute of Physiological Sciences, Okazaki, Japan) for 30 min. After washing in PBS, coverslips were incubated with secondary antibodies (1:1000 dilution) conjugated with Alexa Fluor 488 (Abcam, Cambridge, UK) or Alexa Fluor 546 (Invitrogen, Carlsbad, CA, USA). After washing, the coverslips were mounted onto glass slides with mounting medium (Fluoromount-G; SBA Southern Biotechnology Associates, Inc., Birmingham, AL, USA). Tissues were visualized using a laser scanning microscope (LSM700; Zeiss, Oberkochen, Germany).

4.8. Statistical and Data Analyses

Experimental values are given as the means ± SE of the indicated number of the animals. Comparisons between two groups were made with unpaired or paired Student's *t*-test or the Mann–Whitney test. In all instances, $p < 0.05$ was considered to be statistically significant. The K_m and V_{max} values for the I_{sc} response were determined by fitting the concentration response to the Michaelis–Menten equation using nonlinear regression with GraphPad Prism software (San Diego, CA, USA).

Author Contributions: Conceptualization, H.H. and A.I.; investigation, N.I., M.N., and H.H.; formal analysis, M.N., N.I., W.H., and H.H.; writing, H.H. All authors have read and agreed to the published version of the manuscript.

Funding: This work was supported by JSPS KAKENHI grant number 25282024 (to H.H. and A.I.) and 17K00860 (to H.H. and N.I.). This study was supported in part by grants from the Salt Science Research Foundation grant number 1831 (to H.H. and N.I.). W.H. is a recipient of the Otsuka Toshimi Scholarship Foundation from 2018 to 2020.

Acknowledgments: We thank Sachiko Tsukita and Atsushi Tamura for providing claudin-15 deficient mice.

Conflicts of Interest: The authors declare no conflict of interest. The funders had no role in the design of the study; in the collection, analyses, or interpretation of data; in the writing of the manuscript, or in the decision to publish the results.

Abbreviations

αMDG	α-methyl-D-glucose
G_t	transmural conductance
I_{sc}	short-circuit current
J	flux
V_{te}	transepithelial potential difference
MS	mucosal to serosal
SM	serosal to mucosal
NHE3	Na^+/H^+ exchanger-3 isoform
IBMX	isobutylmethylxanthine
K_m	Michaelis–Menten constant
V_{max}	value of the maximum change
ORS	oral rehydration solution

References

1. Kato, A.; Romero, M.F. Regulation of Electroneutral NaCl Absorption by the Small Intestine. *Annu. Rev. Physiol.* **2011**, *73*, 261–281. [CrossRef] [PubMed]
2. Peerce, B.E.; Wright, E.M. Conformational changes in the intestinal brush border sodium-glucose cotransporter labeled with fluorescein isothiocyanate. *Proc. Natl. Acad. Sci. USA* **1984**, *81*, 2223–2226. [CrossRef] [PubMed]
3. Prasad, P.D.; Wang, H.; Huang, W.; Leibach, F.H.; Ganapathy, V. Cloning of a cDNA encoding the human sodium-dependent vitamin transporter mediating the uptake of pantothenate, biotin and lipoate. *J. Biol. Chem.* **1998**, *273*, 7501–7506. [CrossRef] [PubMed]
4. Yao, S.Y.M.; Muzyka, W.R.; Elliott, J.F.; Cheeseman, C.I.; Young, J.D. Poly(a)+ RNA from the mucosa of rat jejunum induces novel na+-dependent and na+-independent leucine transport activities in in oocytes of xenopus laevis. *Mol. Membr. Biol.* **1994**, *11*, 109–118. [CrossRef]
5. Cordain, L.; Eaton, S.B.; Sebastian, A.; Mann, N.; Lindeberg, S.; Watkins, B.A.; O'Keefe, J.H.; Brand-Miller, J. Origins and evolution of the Western diet: Health implications for the 21st century. *Am. J. Clin. Nutr.* **2005**, *81*, 341–354. [CrossRef]
6. Hediger, M.A.; Coady, M.J.; Ikeda, T.S.; Wright, E.M. Expression cloning and cDNA sequencing of the Na+/glucose co-transporter. *Nature* **1987**, *330*, 379–381. [CrossRef]
7. Mackenzie, B.; Loo, D.D.F.; Wright, E.M. Relationships between Na+/glucose cotransporter (SGLT1) currents and fluxes. *J. Membr. Biol.* **1998**, *162*, 101–106. [CrossRef]
8. Phillips, S.F. Diarrhea: A current view of the pathophysiology. *Gastroenterology* **1972**, *63*, 495–518. [CrossRef]
9. Powell, D.W. Barrier function of epithelia. *Am. J. Physiol.* **1981**, *241*, G275–G288. [CrossRef]
10. Tsukita, S.; Tanaka, H.; Tamura, A. The Claudins: From Tight Junctions to Biological Systems. *Trends Biochem. Sci.* **2019**, *44*, 141–152. [CrossRef]
11. Rahner, C.; Mitic, L.L.; Anderson, J.M. Heterogeneity in expression and subcellular localization of claudins 2, 3, 4, and 5 in the rat liver, pancreas, and gut. *Gastroenterology* **2001**, *120*, 411–422. [CrossRef] [PubMed]
12. Rendón-Huerta, E.; Teresa, F.; Teresa, G.M.; Xochitl, G.-S.; Georgina, A.-F.; Veronica, Z.-Z.; Montaño, L.F. Distribution and Expression Pattern of Claudins 6, 7, and 9 in Diffuse- and Intestinal-Type Gastric Adenocarcinomas. *J. Gastrointest. Cancer* **2010**, *41*, 52–59. [CrossRef] [PubMed]
13. Tamura, A.; Kitano, Y.; Hata, M.; Katsuno, T.; Moriwaki, K.; Sasaki, H.; Hayashi, H.; Suzuki, Y.; Noda, T.; Furuse, M.; et al. Megaintestine in Claudin-15-Deficient Mice. *Gastroenterology* **2008**, *134*, 523–534. [CrossRef] [PubMed]
14. Tamura, A.; Hayashi, H.; Imasato, M.; Yamazaki, Y.; Hagiwara, A.; Wada, M.; Noda, T.; Watanabe, M.; Suzuki, Y.; Tsukita, S. Loss of claudin-15, but not claudin-2, causes Na^+ deficiency and glucose malabsorption in mouse small intestine. *Gastroenterology* **2011**, *140*, 913–923. [CrossRef] [PubMed]
15. Halperin, M.L.; Wolman, S.L.; Greenberg, G.R. Paracellular recirculation of sodium is essential to support nutrient absorption in the gastrointestinal tract: An hypothesis. *Clin. Investig. Med.* **1986**, *9*, 209–211.
16. Binder, H.J.; Brown, I.; Ramakrishna, B.S.; Young, G.P. Oral rehydration therapy in the second decade of the twenty-first century. *Curr. Gastroenterol. Rep.* **2014**, *16*, 376. [CrossRef] [PubMed]

17. Gawenis, L.R.; Stien, X.; Shull, G.E.; Schultheis, P.J.; Woo, A.L.; Walker, N.M.; Clarke, L.L. Intestinal NaCl transport in NHE2 and NHE3 knockout mice. *Am. J. Physiol. Liver Physiol.* **2002**, *282*, G776–G784. [CrossRef]
18. Pappenheimer, J.R.; Reiss, K.Z. Contribution of solvent drag through intercellular junctions to absorption of nutrients by the small intestine of the rat. *J. Membr. Biol.* **1987**, *100*, 123–136. [CrossRef]
19. Lin, R.; Murtazina, R.; Cha, B.; Chakraborty, M.; Sarker, R.; Chen, T.; Lin, Z.; Hogema, B.M.; De Jonge, H.R.; Seidler, U.; et al. D-glucose acts via sodium/glucose cotransporter 1 to increase NHE3 in mouse jejunal brush border by a Na+/H+ exchange regulatory factor 2dependent process. *Gastroenterology* **2011**, *140*, 560–571. [CrossRef]
20. Schwark, J.-R.; Jansen, H.W.; Lang, H.-J.; Krick, W.; Burckhardt, G.; Hropot, M. S3226, a novel inhibitor of Na^+/H^+ exchanger subtype 3 in various cell types. *Pflugers Arch. Eur. J. Physiol.* **1998**, *436*, 797–800. [CrossRef]
21. Halm, D.R.; Dawson, D.C. Control of potassium transport by turtle colon: Role of membrane potential. *Am. J. Physiol.* **1984**, *247*, C26–C32. [CrossRef] [PubMed]
22. Ishizuka, N.; Nakayama, M.; Watanabe, M.; Tajima, H.; Yamauchi, Y.; Ikari, A.; Hayashi, H. Luminal Na^+ homeostasis has an important role in intestinal peptide absorption in vivo. *Am. J. Physiol.* **2018**, *315*, G799–G809. [CrossRef] [PubMed]
23. Frizzell, R.A.; Schultz, S.G. Ionic Conductances of Extracellular Shunt Pathway in Rabbit Ileum. *J. Gen. Physiol.* **1972**, *59*, 318–346. [CrossRef] [PubMed]
24. Field, M. Intestinal ion transport and the pathophysiology of diarrhea Find the latest version: Intestinal ion transport and the pathophysiology of diarrhea. *J. Clin. Investig.* **2003**, *111*, 931–943. [CrossRef]
25. Powell, D.W. Intestinal conductance and permselectivity changes with theophylline and choleragen. *Am. J. Physiol.* **1974**, *227*, 1436–1443. [CrossRef]
26. Gawenis, L.R.; Boyle, K.T.; Palmer, B.A.; Walker, N.M.; Clarke, L.L. Lateral intercellular space volume as a determinant of CFTR-mediated anion secretion across small intestinal mucosa. *Am. J. Physiol. Liver Physiol.* **2004**, *286*, G1015–G1023. [CrossRef]
27. Smith, D.E.; Clémençon, B.; Hediger, M.A. Proton-coupled oligopeptide transporter family SLC15: Physiological, pharmacological and pathological implications. *Mol. Aspects Med.* **2013**, *34*, 323–336. [CrossRef]
28. Ishizuka, N.; Hempstock, W.; Hayashi, H. The Mode of Action of NHE3 Inhibitors in Intestinal Na + Absorption. *Gastroenterol. Med. Res.* **2019**, *4*, 297–299.
29. Uchida, R.; Iwamoto, K.; Nagayama, S.; Miyajima, A.; Okamoto, H.; Ikuta, N.; Fukumi, H.; Terao, K.; Hirota, T. Effect of γ-cyclodextrin inclusion complex on the absorption of R-α-lipoic acid in rats. *Int. J. Mol. Sci.* **2015**, *16*, 10105–10120. [CrossRef]
30. Gorboulev, V.; Schürmann, A.; Vallon, V.; Kipp, H.; Jaschke, A.; Klessen, D.; Friedrich, A.; Scherneck, S.; Rieg, T.; Cunard, R.; et al. Na^+-D-glucose cotransporter SGLT1 is pivotal for intestinal glucose absorption and glucose-dependent incretin secretion. *Diabetes* **2012**, *61*, 187–196. [CrossRef]
31. Yu, A.S.L.; Cheng, M.H.; Angelow, S.; Günzel, D.; Kanzawa, S.A.; Schneeberger, E.E.; Fromm, M.; Coalson, R.D. Molecular Basis for Cation Selectivity in Claudin-2–based Paracellular Pores: Identification of an Electrostatic Interaction Site. *J. Gen. Physiol.* **2009**, *133*, 111–127. [CrossRef] [PubMed]
32. Wada, M.; Tamura, A.; Takahashi, N.; Tsukita, S. Loss of claudins 2 and 15 from mice causes defects in paracellular Na^+ flow and nutrient transport in gut and leads to death from malnutrition. *Gastroenterology* **2013**, *144*, 369–380. [CrossRef] [PubMed]
33. Schultheis, P.J.; Meneton, P.; Riddle, T.M.; Duffy, J.J.; Doetschman, T.; Shull, G.E.; Miller, M.L.; Soleimani, M.; Lorenz, J.N.; Wang, T.; et al. Renal and intestinal absorptive defects in mice lacking the NHE3 Na^+/H^+ exchanger. *Nat. Genet.* **1998**, *19*, 282–285. [CrossRef] [PubMed]
34. Schweinfest, C.W.; Spyropoulos, D.D.; Henderson, K.W.; Kim, J.H.; Chapman, J.M.; Barone, S.; Worrell, R.T.; Wang, Z.; Soleimani, M. slc26a3 (dra)-deficient mice display chloride-losing diarrhea, enhanced colonic proliferation, and distinct up-regulation of ion transporters in the colon. *J. Biol. Chem.* **2006**, *281*, 37962–37971. [CrossRef]
35. Duffey, M.E.; Hainau, B.; Ho, S.; Bentzel, C.J. Regulation of epithelial tight junction permeability by cyclic AMP. *Nature* **1981**, *294*, 451–453. [CrossRef]
36. Field, M.; Fromm, D.; al-Awqati, Q.; Greenough, W.B. Effect of cholera enterotoxin on Ion transport across isolated ileal mucosa. *J. Clin. Investig.* **1972**, *51*, 796–804. [CrossRef]

37. Duggan, C.; Fontaine, O.; Pierce, N.F.; Glass, R.I.; Mahalanabis, D.; Alam, N.H.; Bhan, M.K.; Santosham, M. Scientific Rationale for a Change in the Composition of Oral Rehydration Solution. *JAMA* **2004**, *291*, 2628–2631. [CrossRef]
38. Singh, A.K.; Amlal, H.; Haas, P.J.; Dringenberg, U.; Fussell, S.; Barone, S.L.; Engelhardt, R.; Zuo, J.; Seidler, U.; Soleimani, M. Fructose-induced hypertension: Essential role of chloride and fructose absorbing transporters PAT1 and Glut5. *Kidney Int.* **2008**, *74*, 438–447. [CrossRef]
39. Fayad, I.M.; Kamel, M.; Hirschhorn, N.; Abu-Zikry, M. Hypernatraemia surveillance during a national diarrhoeal diseases control project in Egypt. *Lancet* **1992**, *339*, 389–393. [CrossRef]

MDPI
St. Alban-Anlage 66
4052 Basel
Switzerland
Tel. +41 61 683 77 34
Fax +41 61 302 89 18
www.mdpi.com

International Journal of Molecular Sciences Editorial Office
E-mail: ijms@mdpi.com
www.mdpi.com/journal/ijms

CPSIA information can be obtained
at www.ICGtesting.com
Printed in the USA
LVHW051806150422
716314LV00006B/380

9 783036 519319